NEUROSCIENCE RESEARCH PROGRESS

PRENATAL ALCOHOL EXPOSURE AND ITS EFFECTS ON HIPPOCAMPAL ANATOMY AND FUNCTION

NEUROSCIENCE RESEARCH PROGRESS

Additional books in this series can be found on Nova's website under theSeries tab.

Additional E-books in this series can be found on Nova's website under the E-books tab.

NEUROSCIENCE RESEARCH PROGRESS

PRENATAL ALCOHOL EXPOSURE AND ITS EFFECTS ON HIPPOCAMPAL ANATOMY AND FUNCTION

JOANNA H. SLIWOWSKA

Nova Science Publishers, Inc.
New York

For permission to use material from this book please contact us:
Telephone 631-231-7269; Fax 631-231-8175
Web Site: http://www.novapublishers.com

Library of Congress Cataloging-in-Publication Data

Sliwowska, Joanna H.
Prenatal alcohol exposure and its effects on hippocampal anatomy and function / Joanna H. Sliwowska.
p. ; cm.
Includes bibliographical references and index.
ISBN 978-1-61668-922-3 (softcover)
1. Fetal alcohol syndrome--Pathophysiology. 2. Hippocampus (Brain)--Toxicology. 3. Hippocampus (Brain)--Pathophysiology. I. Title.
[DNLM: 1. Hippocampus--drug effects. 2. Ethanol--adverse effects. 3. Prenatal Exposure Delayed Effects. WL 314 S633p 2010]
RG629.F45S45 2010 618.3'268--dc22- 2010016715

Published by Nova Science Publishers, Inc. † New York

Contents

Preface

Over the years several individuals and institutions have helped in various ways with the creation of this book. I am especially grateful to Dr. Joanne Weinberg who introduced me to the field of prenatal alcohol exposure and created a supportive environment in which I was able to gain knowledge and experience. I am also very fortune to have had the opportunity to collaborate with Dr. LiisaGalea, an expert in the field of adult hippocampal neurogenesis. I would also like to express my thanks to all members of Weinberg and Galea laboratories for their inspiration and help these past years. My special thank you to Tamara Bodnar for her excellent editorial help during the process of writingthis book. I would also like to thank Drs. McEwen, Morris, Sapolsky, Plotsky, Herman, and Miller for the inspirations I have gained from reading their papers, which has greatly facilitated my writing of this book. I would also like to express my gratitude to Drs. Szyfter, Skrzypczak, Nässel, Tublitz, Lehman, Goodman, Karsch, Coolen and Viau for their assistance in my journey through the field of neuroendocrinology. The creation of this book would not have been possible without support from the following institutions: the Adam Mickiewicz University, Poznań, Poland; Poznań University of Life Sciences, Poznań, Poland; Stockholm University, Sweden; Oregon University, Eugene, OR, USA; The University of Cincinnati, Cincinnati, OH, USA and The University of British Columbia, Vancouver, BC, Canada, where I have gained knowledge and training throughout my career. My work would also not have been possible without generous funding from the governments of Poland (KBN), the Sweden (Swedish Institute), the USA (NIH) and Canadian (CIHR, IMPART, HELP, BlumaTischler Fellowship).

The research presented in this book was funded by following fellowship and grants: BlumaTischler Fellowship and CIHR (IMPART) to Dr. Joanna H.

Sliwowska; R37AA07789 NIH/NIAA to Dr. Joanne Weinberg; 06-3844 BC Ministry of Children and Family Development (through theUBC Human Early Learning Partnership) to Drs. Joanne Weinberg and Liisa Galea.

Finally, I would like to thank my husband and my children for creating a supportive environment in which I have been able to develop my passion for neuroscience. Thanks to my family for understanding that science requires great sacrifices. Great thanks also to my parents and my sister for all of their support as it is the support of my family that has made this book possible.

The part of this book has appeared previously in the following publications: Śliwowska J. H. (in press) Long-term effects of prenatal alcohol exposure on the hippocampal anatomy and functions In: Hippocampus: Anatomy Functions and Neurobiology. Ed: Ambroise Gärtner and Dener Frantz. Nova Science Publisher, and Śliwowska J. H., Zhang X., Weinberg J. (2006) Prenatal ethanol exposure and fetal programming: implications for endocrine and immune development and long-term health. p. 153-181. In: Brain development. Normal Processes and Effects of Alcohol and Nicotine Ed. Michael W. Miller. Oxford University Press.

Author's Contact Information

Joanna H. Sliwowska , Ph.D.
Department of Histology and Embryology
Institute of Zoology
Poznan University of Life Sciences
ul. Wojska Polskiego 71c
60-625 Poznan, Poland
phone: +48 61 848 7627

Organization and Contents

The aim of this book is to provide evidence in support of the hypothesis that prenatal alcohol/ethanol exposure (PAE) interferes with normal development and function of the hippocampus. In this book, the hippocampus will be viewed as a target for early (prenatal) aversive events, such as PAE. Early life events are complex and interact with genetic factors in a manner which is not yet fully understood but which can profoundly change the structure and function of the hippocampus.This is not surprising as the hippocampus plays a crucial role not only in learning, memory storage and retrieval but also in controlling the stress response.

To achieve the above goal, this book is organized into five main chapters. First, Fetal Alcohol Spectrum Disorder (FASD) with be presented from a historical perspective in the chapter entitled: Fetal Alcohol Spectrum Disorder (FASD): A Historical Perspective. Next, the hippocampus, will be introduced in the chapter entitled: Neurobiology, Anatomy and Development of the Hippocampus. These two chapters together will provide the foundation to allow for subsequent exploration of the damage to the hippocampus associated with prenatal alcohol consumption in the chapter entitled: Hippocampus and Prenatal Alcohol Exposure. Next, the fourth chapter entitled: Can We Prevent or Reverse the Effects of Prenatal Alcohol Exposure on the Hippocampus? Intervention, Prevention and Implication will focus on application of the knowledge gained from the aforementioned studies. Finally, this book will end with the chapter entitled: General Conclusion.

I hope that readers are able to find, in the pages of this book, a wide array of anatomical, histological, physiological and behavioral support of the hypothesis that prenatal alcohol/ethanol exposure interferes with normal development and function of the hippocampus. I also hope that readers will start to appreciate that emerging therapeutic strategies provide us with hope for improving the lives of individuals experiencing the devastating and long-term effects of *in utero* alcohol exposure.

Chapter I

Fetal Alcohol Spectrum Disorder (FASD): A Historical Perspective

For decades, people have been cautioned as to the danger of alcohol use and abuse during pregnancy. The Bible is most likely one of the first written sources, which refers to the effects of prenatal alcohol exposure on fetal development. In the Old Testament, the Book of Judges introduces Samson at the time of his conception. Samson's parents had given up all hope of having children. Samson's mother is deep in despair when an angel appears and tells her that she is pregnant and will bear a son. The angel also instructs her to refrain from drinking during her pregnancy: *"Thou shalt conceive, and bear a son. Nowtherefore, beware, I pray thee, and drink not wine nor strong drink"* (Judges 13:3-4). Later, we find another reference to drinking during conception in the text of the great philosopher Plato: *[A man] " steeped in wine...is clumsy and bad at sowing seed, and is thus likely to beget unstable and untrusty offspring, crooked in form and character"*/Abel 1997, Abel 1999, Plato (reprint 1952)/. The above quotations are, however, taken out of context and are difficult to interpret without the historical and cultural context from the past. In depth studies by Davis (Davis 1980) and Abel (Abel 1997, Abel 1999) shed light on the possible meanings of these quotations and they conclude that people from that time may not have been aware of the potential dangers of alcohol on the unborn child /for a review see (Abel 1997, Abel 1999)/. Much later, multiple resources emerged with information as to the effects of alcohol on the fetusand this coincided with the so called "gin epidemic". Indeed, in

England between 1720 and 1750, there are reports of decreased birth rates and increased rates of stillbirths and infant mortality. Interestingly, art, in addition to written records, indicate possible historical awareness as to the detrimental effects of alcohol on the fetus. The 18th century painter William Hogarth, in his 1751 painting entitled *Gin Lane,* presents the poverty-stricken area to the north of Covent Garden in London. In this painting, a half-naked drunken woman fails to notice that her child is falling to a certain death. A number of medical historians have found that the infant falling from the woman'sarms shows facial features characteristic of what is now called Fetal Alcohol Syndrome (FAS). Whether the painter was aware of alcohol's prenatal effects or whether experts were biased in their description based on current knowledge of FAS remains unknown (Abel 2001).

It was not until 1973 that the disorder resulting from high maternal alcohol consumption was termed FAS by Jones and Smith (Jones & Smith 1973). These scientists examined eight children born to alcoholic mothers and found that they all had a very similar pattern of craniofacial malformations. Later, it was shown that prenatal exposure to high levels of alcohol can result in central nervous system dysfunction, growth deficiencies and a specific facial dysmorphology – three of the key diagnostic criteria for FAS (Figure 1). However, FAS is at the extreme end of the spectrum of deficits that result from prenatal alcohol exposure. Because it has been recognized that exposed individuals may have some, but not all, of the characteristics of FAS, the term Fetal Alcohol Spectrum Disorder (FASD) was coined and is used as an umbrella term covering the wide range of outcomes associated with PAE (Sokol et al 2003).

Children prenatally exposed to alcohol have primary deficits in cognition, communication, learning, memory and behavior, including high levels of maladaptive behaviors (Olsen et al 1998, Streissguth et al 1996, Streissguth et al 2004). Among the most common secondary deficits reported in children and adults with FASD are mental illness, and in particular, depression and anxiety disorders (Famy et al 1998, O'Connor & Paley 2006, Streissguth et al 1996, Streissguth et al 2004).

Despite overwhelming evidence as to the harmful effects of alcohol on the fetus, the incidence of FAS remains high. The prevalence rate of FAS was 0.5 to 2 cases per 1,000 births and as high as 10 cases per 1,000 births for FASD in the United States during the 1980s and 1990s (May & Gossage 2001).

Of particular relevance to this book, is the finding that the hippocampus is profoundly susceptible to the teratogenic effects of PAE (Berman & Hannigan 2000, West et al 1981).

Craniofacial features associated with fetal alcohol syndrome

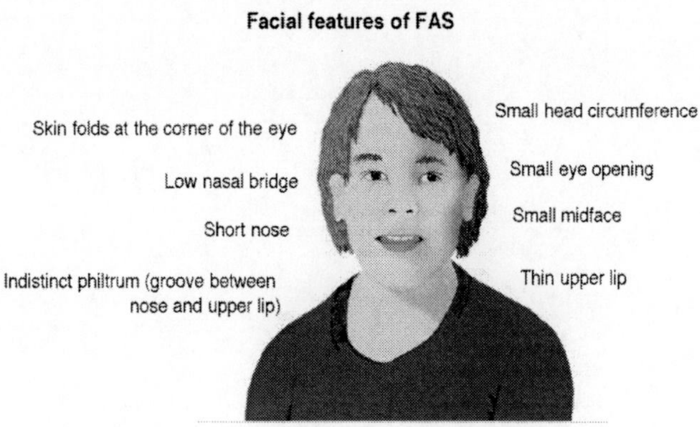

A characteristic pattern of mild facial anomalies, including small eye openings (i.e., short palpebral fissures), a thin upper lip, or flattened ridges between the base of the nose and the upper lip (i.e., a flattened philtrum) associated with FAS.

Figure 1. Craniofacial features associated with Fetal Alcohol Syndrome (FAS). (Source: Reprinted from Warren et al., (2001) with permission from the NIAAA)

Chapter II

Neurobiology, Anatomy and Development of the Hippocampus

1. Neurobiology of the Hippocampus: Historical Perspective and Initial Connections between Alcohol Consumption and Hippocampal Damage

This chapter has three main goals: First, is to provide an overview of important historically discoveries that lead to the initial elucidation of the functions of the hippocampus. Second, is to emphasize the development and importance of new techniques, which have allowed for in-depth studies of the hippocampus. Finally, is to discuss evidence for the connection between alcohol and hippocampal damage. As great conceptual advances in science are often based on significant technical advances, it is my aim to provide evidence for their interrelationship throught this chapter.

The hippocampus has a rather striking appearance, which astonished ancient anatomists. It has an elegant, curved structure, which, when seen together with its contralateral half, strongly resembles the coiled horns of a ram (Figure 2). Thus, due its shape, ancient scholars named the hippocampus *cornu ammonium* (*Latin for horn of ram*). This name is used today to denote the subfields of the hippocampus: CA1 (*cornuammonis*), CA2 and CA3 (Figure 3). In 1587, the Italian anatomist Julius Cesear Arantius was the first to coin the name "hippocampus", as this brain structure resembles the sea horse, a tropical fish, as *hippos* is Greek for horse and *kampos* means sea monster (Per Andersen 2007) (Figure 4). Later, the Italian scientist, Camillo Golgi (1843–1926) invented a new technique, greatly contributing to the advancement of the field of hipppocampal neuroanatomy. Using the novel technique called the black reaction (now referred to as the Golgi method), Golgi was ableto visualize individual nerve cells in unprecedented detail /see the translation of Golgi's orginal paper first published in 1883 (Golgi et al 2001)/:

> "The pes Hippocampi major is a region of the cerebrum that presents a very complex structure. There is a great deal of interest in studying this structure because determining the exact shape of the cells that form it, and the course and organization of its nerve fiber bundles, may shed light on its function, which remains quite obscure".

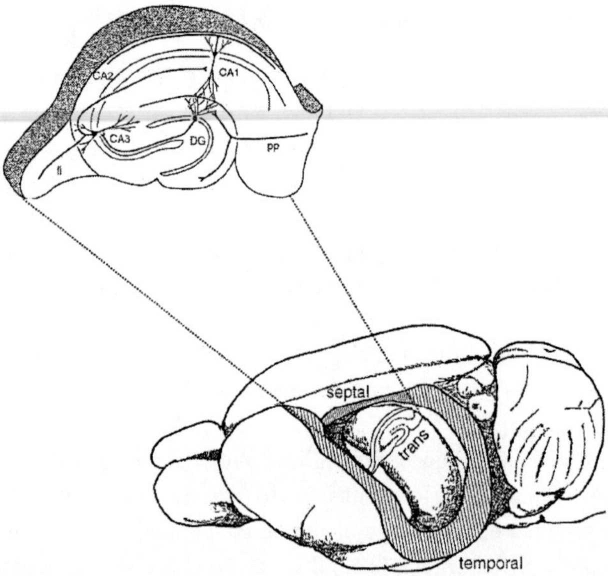

Figure 2. Line drawing of the rat brain shows septotemporaral and transverse axes of the hippocampal formation. (Source: Reprinted from: Amaral DLP et al., (2007) with permission from Oxford University Press).

This discovery paved the way for the later development of new hypotheses as to the anatomical organization and function of the nervous system (Van Gijn 2001). Among his numerous contributions to our understanding of cerebral gross anatomy, Golgi also discovered that the dentate gyrus and the hippocampus form two very distinct gyri (Golgi et al 2001). For his work on the structure of the nervous system, Golgi shared the 1906 Nobel Prize with another great scientist Santiago Ramón y Cajal (for detailed information see the Nobel Foundation webpage: http://nobelprize.org/nobel_prizes/medicine/articles/grant/index.html.

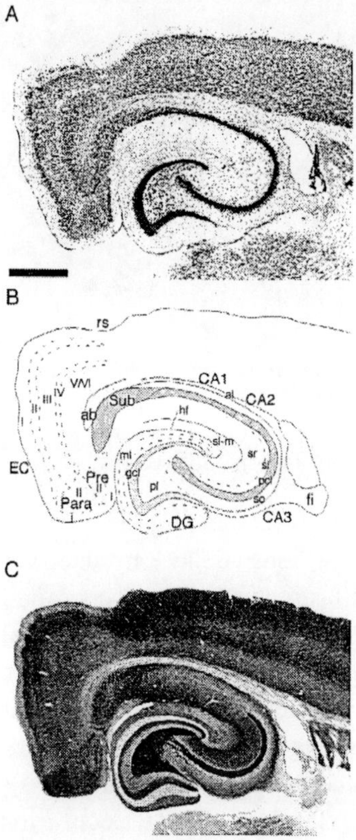

Figure 3. Horizontal section through the rat hippocampus. (A) Nissel-stained section. (B) Line drawing shows various regions, layers, and fiber pathways. (C) Timm's sulfide silver-stained section. In (C) three bands in molecular layer in the DR are visible. ab – angular bundle; al – alveus; CA1, CA2, CA3 –subfields of the hippocampus; DG – dentate gyrus; EC – entorhinal cortex; fi – fimbria; gcl – granule cell layer of the dentate gyrus; hf – hippocampal fissure; ml – molecular layer of the dentate gyrus; Para - parasubiculum ; Pre – presubiculum; pcl – pyramidal layer of the hippocampus; pl – polymorphic layer of the dentate gyrus; sl – stratum lucidum of CA3; sr – stratum radiatum of the hippocampus; sl-m – striatum locunosum moleculare of the hippocampus. Roman numerals – cortical layers. Bar A = 500 μm and applies to all panels. (Source: Reprinted from: Amaral DLP et al. (2007) with permission from Oxford University Press).

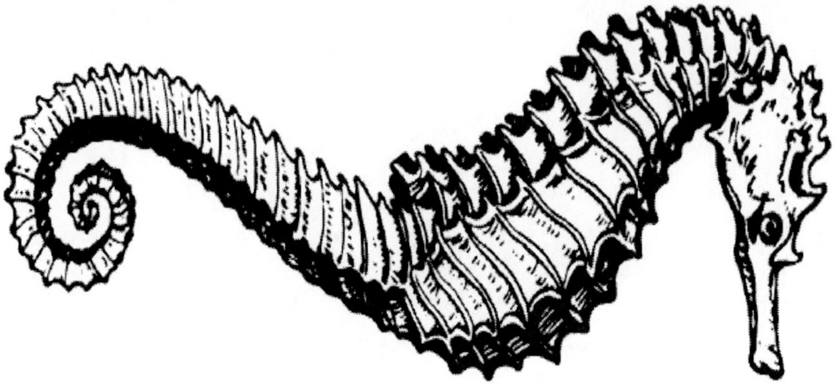

Figure 4. Drawing of the sea horse to which the shape of the hippocampus has been compared (see Figures. 2 and 3). (Adopted from: Neurobiology of the Hippocampus. Ed. W. Seifert, Academic Press, Inc, Source: Gensner's figure of a hippocampus. Hist. animal. Lib. IV De piscium nat., Tiguri, 1558, p. 491).

Despite the increased understanding as to the neuroanatomy of the hippocampus, there was a long delay in determining its function. The suspected roles of this brain structure were diverse and it was considered to be: part of the olfactory system, essential for emotional behavior, controlling attention and finally also involved in memory /see (Per Andersen 2007)/. Of particular interest, the evidence for the role of the hippocampus in memory came from studying the effects of heavy drinking. In 1881, Carl Wernicke first described three cases of alcoholism with the patients all experiencing paralysis of eye movements, ataxia and mental confusion. All three patients subsequently died and *postmortem* studies of their brains revealed punctate hemorrhages affecting the grey matter around the third and fourth ventricles near the aqueduct of Sylvius. At this time, Wernicke believed that the hemorrhages were the result of inflammation. Several years later, independent studies performed by the Russian psychiatrist Sergei S. Korsakov, described a similar condition, with the main symptom being memory deficits. In 1900, the Russian neurologist, Vladimir Bekhterev described two patients experiencing prominent memory deficits and with autopsy revealing softening of the hippocampus and neighboring cortical areas on both sides of the brain. Thus, studying the brains of patients with alcohol-associated damaged (appropriately named the Wernicke-Korsakov syndrome) provided the first piece of evidence that the hippocampus is critically involved in memory formation /for a recent review of the literature see (Kopelman et al 2009)/. Improved understanding of the function of the hippocampus was further facilitated by studying the case of

Henry Molaison, better known in the scientific literature simply as H.M. This man was perhaps the most famous patient in all of brain science during the 20th century. Henry Molaison was born in 1926 and suffered from epileptic seizures since childhood. His overall prognosis being poor, doctors decided to operate on his brain. In 1953 he underwent an experimental operation and the part of his brain believed to be causing the seizures was removed. The operation did succeed in reducing seizure activity, however, he paid a high price as doctors removed a piece of the temporal lobes from both sides of his brain, including most of the hippocampus, amygdala, and nearby parahippocampalgyrus. As a result of this surgery, H.M. could not form new memories lasting more than 20 to 30 seconds. Thus, at the age of 27, Molaison was frozen in time (Miller 2009). His condition was akin to severe amnesia and his case was studied extensively by numerous scientists, resulting in a greater understanding as to howmemories are formed in the brain /see e.g. (Corkin et al 1997, Miller 2009, Scoville & Milner 1957, Squire & Zola-Morgan 1991)/. Molaison forgot names, places, events and faces almost immediately. A half hour after H.M. had lunch, he could not recall what he had eaten, or even thathe had eaten at all. If someone were to ask him a question, he could not remember what he was being asked, even if the question was posed just minutes prior. Surprisingly, however, Molaison easily recalled events that occurred prior to his operation (Scoville & Milner 1957). Molaison could also learn and remember new skills, learn and retain new facts and thus retained what researchers now call declarative memory. Following his surgery, his reflection was a constant surprise as he was only capable of remembering what he looked like as a young man. H.M. died at age 82 of respiratory pneumonia and generously donated his brain to science. In 2009, a large project was launched, beginning with slicing of H.M's brain at the University of California, San Diego. Dr. Jacopo Annese, a neuroanatomist and the principal investigator of this project, plans to create an open-access digital brain librarywith the first contribution being the postmortem analysis and detailed digitization of H.M.'s brain. In addition, this information is complemented by high-resolution MRI scans of H.M's brain (Miller 2009). Clearly, Molaison's case has lead to, and continues to lead to, the advancement of memory research. The most significant contributions include the discovery that there are different types of memory, each dependent on specific brain regions and the concept of memory consolidation whereby new memories formed by the hippocampus are later archived in the cerebral cortex for long-term storage (Miller 2009).

2. Hippocampal Neuroanatomy

Before moving into a discussion as to the effects of alcohol on the hippocampus, the neuroanatomy of this brain structure must be described.This chapter will introduce the anatomical terminology that will be used throughout this book as well as provide background knowledge as to the neuronal organization of the hippocampus and its intrinsic connections, all of which is crucial in order to understand the functions of the hippocampus.

A sticking feature of the hippocampus, when stained and examined under the microscope, is the relatively simple organization of the principal cell layers and the highly organized laminar distribution of many of its inputs (Amaral D 2007). However, despite the relatively long neuroanatomical history of this brain structure (having been described for more than a century), its nomenclature has yet to be formalized. In this book, the hippocampus will be viewed as one of several related brain regions that together comprise the functional system called the hippocampal formation.The term hippocampus will refer to the hippocampus proper, which consists of three subdivisions: CA1, CA2 and CA3. The hippocampal formation also includes other regions such as the dentate gyrus (DG), subiculum, presubiculum, and entorhinal cortex (Figures 3,5). The DG is a region of critical importance for hippocampal neurogenesis, which will be the focus of section ten in chapter three. The DG is comprised of three layers: the molecular layer (relatively cell-free), the granular cell layer, and the polymorphic cell layer. The granular and molecular cell layers form a V- or U-shaped structure (Figures 3,6).

One of the major characteristics of the hippocampal formation is that it receives highly processed sensory information from a variety of neocortical sources. Axons from cells of the entorhinal cortex project to the dentate gyrus and these projections form part of the major hippocampal input pathway called the perforant pathway. Cells in the DG, called granule cells, give rise to axons, called mossy fibers that connect with pyramidal cells of the CA3 field of the hippocampus. The cells of CA3, in turn, send their axons, known as Schaffer collaterals, to the CA1 hippocampal field. Next, cells from the CA1 field project to the subiculum (Amaral D 2007; Figure 5).

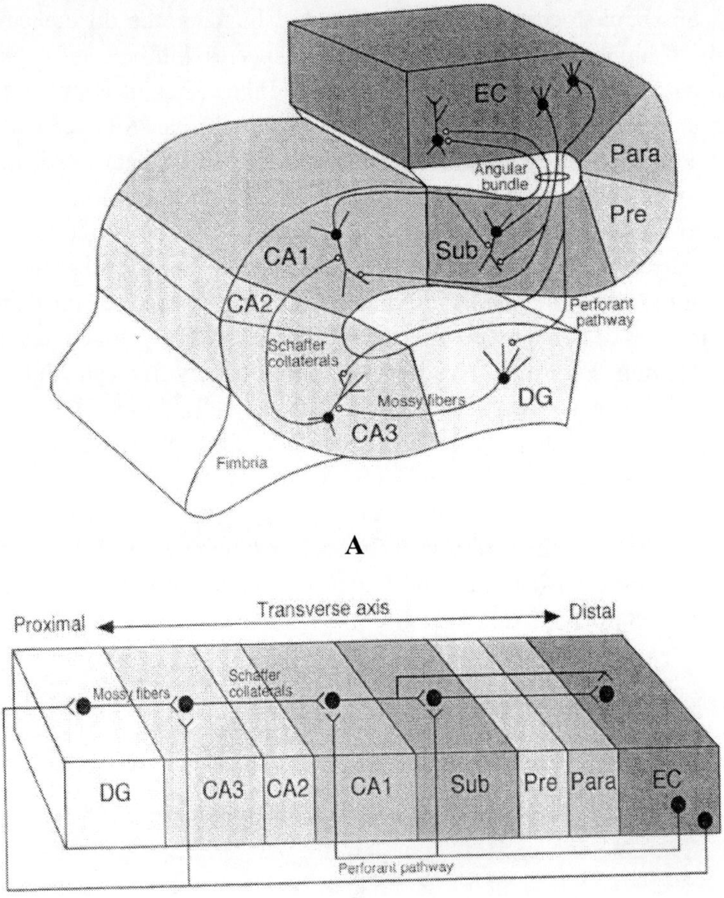

Figure 5. Neuronal projections in the hippocampal formation. (A) Neurons in layer II of the entorhinal cortex project to the dentate gyrus and CA3 field of the hippocampus. Neurons in layer III of the entorhinal cortex project to the CA1 of the hippocampus and the subiculum. The granule cells of the dentate gyrus project to the CA3 field of the hippocampus via mossy fibers projections. Pyramidal neurons in the CA3 field of the hippocampus project to CA1 via Schaffer collaterals. Pyramidal cells in CA1 project to the subiculum. Both CA1 and the subiculum project back to the deep layers of the entorhinal cortex (B). Projections along the transverse axis of the hippocampus. Dente gyrus is located proximally and the entorhinal cortex distally. DG – dentate gyrus, CA1, CA2, CA3 – subfields of the hippocampus, EC - entorhinal cortex, Sub – subiculum. (Source: Reprinted from: Amaral DLP et al., (2007) with permission from Oxford University Press).

As this book focuses mainly on rats and humans, the differences in the anatomy of hippocampus between these two species will be briefly discussed. The rationale for focussing on the rodent and human hippocampus is twofold. Firstly, the purpose of this book is to examine the effects of prenatal alcohol exposure on the hippocampus and this relies on the rodent animal model of PAE as well human studies of FASD/FAS. Another important reason for focusing on the rodent hippocampus (the rat in particular) is that the majority of the current neuroanatomical data has been obtained through studies involving rodents. The main structural difference between the hippocampus of the rat and that of humans relates to the thickness of the pyramidal cell layer in the CA1 region (Figure 6). This layer is approximately five cells thick in rats, whereas in humans it can be more than thirty cells thick. The other main difference is in the enterhinal cortex, which in rats is typically divided into two main subdivisions, but in humans this region is divided into between eight and twenty seven subdivisions (the exact number varying between sources) (Amaral D 2007). There are also differences in the pattern of connectivity of the hippocampus between rats and humans, a topic that will not be discussed further /for details see (Amaral D 2007)/.

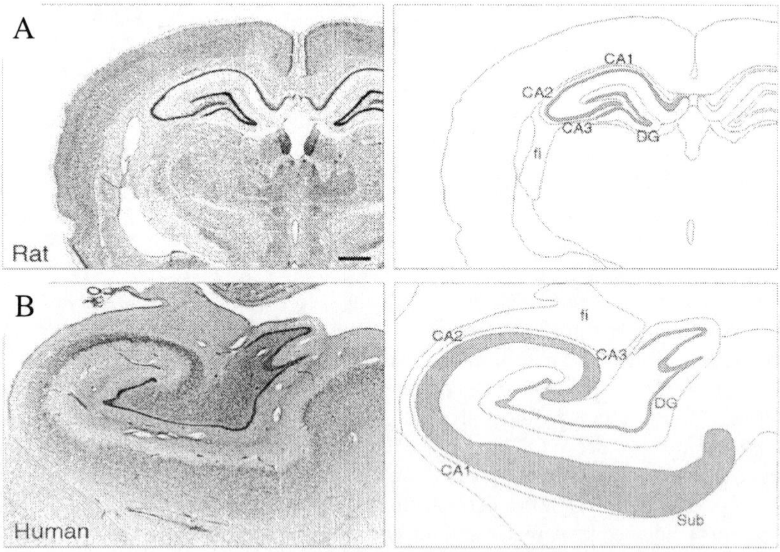

Figure 6. Nissel-stained sections and line drawings illustrating the general organization and similarities of the subdivisions of the hippocampal formation in the rat (A) and human (B). Bar in A=1 mm and applies to all panels. (Reprinted and modified from from: Amaral DLP et al., (2007) with permission from Oxford University Press).

3. Morphological Development of the Hippocampus

An understanding of the development of the hippocampus is required in order to study the effects of prenatal alcohol exposure on the hippocampus. Thus, the goal of this chapter is to describe the morphological development of this brain structure, setting the stage for further discussion as to alcohol's effects at the level of the hippocampus. An in depth examination of the morphological development of the hippocampus is provided by Frotscher and Seress (Frotscher & Seress 2007) with a brief summary of pertinent information included below.

The pyramidal cell layer of the hippocampus in rodents and humans is formed quite early during development. Pyramidal neurons of the hippocampus are generated between embryonic day (E) 10 and 18 in the mouse (Angevine 1965) and between E 16 and 21 in the rat (Bayer 1980). Pregnancy is 19 and 21 days in mice and rats, respectively. In humans, the pyramidal cell layer is formed during the first half of pregnancy (Arnold & Trojanowski 1996). Generation of the granule cell layer in the mouse hippocampus starts at approximately the same time as formation of the first pyramidal cells (on E 10) (Angevine 1965). The generation of granular cells, however, lasts much longer than that of pyramidal cells and continues long into the postnatal period and into adulthood. In the rat, first granular cells of the DG are generated on E 17 and this process persists throughout adult life (Bayer 1980). Thus, the time span of granule cell generation in rodents is about three times longer than that of pyramidal cells. In humans, formation of granule cells lasts for more than 30 weeks and begins during the 13th embryonic week and also continues into adulthood (Eriksson et al 1998, Humphrey 1967, Seress et al 2001). Postmitotic granule cells migrate from the ventricular germinal layer to the DG that surrounds the tip of the CA3 region of the hippocampus. The dentate gyrus consists of two blades of cells and the tip of the CA3 region borders the hilus of dentate gyrus (Frotscher & Seress 2007). After migration from the ventricular germinal layer, stem cells form a secondary germinative layer in the hilus and further proliferation occurs as they move to the granule cell layer of the dentate gyrus. It is important to mention that during the embryonic period, both routes are used; however, during the prenatal period the latter route is used more commonly (Frotscher & Seress 2007).

4. The Hippocampus Is a Very Plastic Brain Structure. "You Can Teach Old Dog New Tricks"

"Plasticity" is defined as the capacity for being molded or altered and this term has also been employed in neuroscience as neuronal plasticity.

The hippocampus is a very plastic brain structure, capable not only of substantial reorganization after damage but also of dramatic structural changes when intact, under normal conditions. These changes in the hippocampus occur in the form of dendritic extensions and retractions, changes in dendritic spine morphology (small protrusions on the dendrites of principal neurons), generation of new neurons in adulthood (neurogenesis), as well as formation and elimination of synapses.The above-mentioned changes are examples of structural plasticity. The term "synaptic plasticity" was coined by the Polish neurophysiologist and psychologist JerzyKonorski to describe the persistent, activity driven changes in synaptic efficacy assumed to form the basis of information storage in the brain (Konorski 1948). Later, two forms of synaptic plasticity were discovered, known as long-term potentiation (LTP) and long-term depression (LTD), and they are thought to play important functional roles in the processes of learning and memory.

Based on the evidence presented above, the hippocampus should be viewed as being a dynamic structure undergoing continuous rearrangement. Factors that have been shown to affect neuronal plasticity in the hippocampus include: ovarian steroids, adrenal steroids, stress, environmental enrichment and alcohol and these will be discussed in later chapters.

Chapter III

The Hippocampus and Prenatal Alcohol Exposure

In previous sections, general anatomy, development and neurobiology, of the hippocampus are discussed. In contrast, this chapter will focus on the negative effects of alcohol on hippocampal structure and function, in particular, prenatal ethanol exposure. It is important to note that the main emphasis will be on long-term (or life-long) effects of PAE, effects that persist into adulthood. First, animal models of PAE will be discussed as they have uncovered information of critical importance to alcohol's effect on the hippocampus. Next, human studies involving magnetic resonance imaging (MRI) will be presented, followed by a discussion of hippocampal-dependent behavioral tests, which highlight some of the effects of prenatal ethanol exposure.

1. Animal Models of Ethanol Exposure: Methods of Ethanol Administration

Animal models serve a crucial role in studying the effects of ethanol exposure on various organs, including brain. They allow for the tight control of factors that cannot be controlled for in human studies, such as dose, pattern, timing and duration of alcohol exposure relative to fetal development, multi-drug use and sample size /for reviews see: (Cudd 2005, Ponnappa & Rubin

2000, Tabakoff & Hoffman 2000, West & Goodlett 1990)/. One of the most widely used animal models for studying prenatal ethanol exposure is the rat.The advantage of using this model is that there exists a wealth of research and literature in a wide range of areas (e.g. anatomy, physiology) that has performed on the rat, including well-established behavioral tasks.

Administration of ethanol in drinking water may seem like the simplest way in which to administer ethanol to laboratory animals, however, animals are generally averse to the taste of ethanol. Thus, using this technique, dehydration resulting from insufficient fluid intake and nutritional imbalance often occurs. Additionally, using this paradigm, only low blood alcohol levels (BALs) can be achieved. Thus, a good alternative appears to be a feeding paradigm in which a liquid ethanol diet is provided as the sole source of nutrition and fluids and this is the method of choice used in our laboratory. This method of ethanol administration is also nonstressful and provides adequate nutrition to the pregnant dams /for a review see (Lieber & DeCarli 1989)/. However, a drawback to the liquid ethanol diet is that very high BALs are difficult to achieve. Additionally, due to reduced food intake typical for animals on the liquid ethanol diet compared to *ad libitum-fed* control animals, there is the need to introduce an additional control group. Thus,a pair-fed (PF) nutritional control group is added to all studies involving liquid ethanol diets.The pair-fed (PF) animals are offered a liquid control diet with maltose-dextrin isocalorically substituted for ethanol and their intake is matched to the amount consumed by an ethanol-treated partner (g/kg body weight/gestation day). However, it is also important to note that pair-feeding is in many ways a treatment in itself as the pair-feeding procedure may constitute a mild form of prenatal stress (Gallo & Weinberg 1981, Weinberg 1984, Vieau et al., 2007). In contrast to ethanol consuming dams who receive *ad libitum* access to their diet throughout the 24-h period, pair-fed dams get a reduced ration of food and typically consume their entire daily portion by a few hours post food presentation. Thus, these PF animals are hungry and without food for a large part of the 24-hours period. Another drawback of pair-feeding is the inability to control for ethanol's effects on absorption and utilization of nutrients.

An alternative to the liquid ethanol diet is intragastric intubation, which consists of inserting a feeding tube directly into the stomach.This method has many advantages including: allowing for aconsistent dose of ethanol to be administered to all animals, the achievement of high BALs and the ability to control for the timing of ethanol administration. However, the drawback is the high mortality rate due to the stressful nature of this route of ethanol administration. Additionally, this method involves handling of the dam, which could confound the results. Alcohol can also be administered acutely via intraperitoneal injections. In spite of the fact that this method gives rise to high BALs and that one can control for the dose of ethanol, this intraperitoneal injection method is also very stressful and is not directly comparable to human ingestion of alcohol. Another method of ethanol exposure is the ethanol inhalation vapor method, which is relatively nonstressful and allows for the achievement of high BALs. This method also eliminates the nutritional issue and need for the pair-fed group as the digestive system is bypassed and ethanol exposed animals, when removed from the vapor chamber, eat well and do not differ in body weight compared to control animals. On the other hand, in human FAS studies, growth deficiencies related to decreased maternal caloric intake are a constant finding, and one of the features of this disease. Another drawback to the ethanol inhalation vapor method is that it results in sustained high BALs, which do not mimic typical human alcohol consumption in which alcohol levels vary through the day. Lastly, as previously mentioned, using this method, the alcohol does not pass through the digestive system, as it does in the human case. As humans ingest alcohol, some of the teratogenic effects of alcohol may be related to the effects of alcohol on food intake and/or nutrient absorption and this cannot be modeled using the vapor method.

Thus, in spite of the drawbacks of the PF group, the liquid ethanol diet is the method of ethanol administration of choice in my studies. Importantly, this method is non-stressful, which is critical when studying the effects of ethanol on the hypothalamic-pituitary-adrenal (HPA) or stress axis function (see section eight, chapter three). It is also important to mention that this method gives rise to moderate BALs, therefore the PAE rats do not display the characteristic features of FAS and thus this method does not model FAS but rather alcohol-related birth deficits (ARBDs).

In addition to the significant benefits of using animal models to study the effects of alcohol exposure, the development of new imaging techniques, such as Magnetic Resonanse Imaging (MRI), are proving to be very valuable in understanding the way in which alcohol cause hippocampal damage.

In summary, PAE animals have the following alterations: excess CORT, an imbalance in hippocampal MR- and GR- receptor levels and impaired negative feedback of the HPA axis. All of the aforementioned changes may contribute to hippocampal damage and to the cognitive impairments reported in animal models of prenatal ethanol exposure and possibly in children with FASD.

9. Serotonergic Involvement in Programming of the HPA Axis: Alterations in the Serotonergic System in Animals Prenatally Exposed to Ethanol

Serotonin, or 5-hydroxytryptamine (5-HT), is known to modulate mood, emotion, sleep and appetite and thus is implicated in the control of numerous behavioral and physiological functions. Modulation of the HPA axis is one of the important physiological functions of 5-HT (Lowry 2002). Thus, not surprisingly, functionning of the serotonergic system is found to be altered in a wide range of conditions and disorders including alcoholism, anxiety, depression, suicide and insomnia (Heinz et al 2001, Lopez et al 1998, Lopez et al 1997, Thase 2006, Tyrer & Baldwin 2006).

The ascending serotonergic innervations of hippocampal neurons arise in the midbrain raphe nuclei and provide a route by which the 5-HT system may act to regulate HPA function. Thus, the hippocampus, where MR, GR,5-HT_{1A} and 5-HT_7 receptors are particularly abundant, represents a unique anatomical environment in which to study the interplay between the serotonergic and HPA systems (Lopez et al 1998).

There is a growing body of evidence suggesting the involvement of the serotonergic system in programming of the HPA axis and several elegant studies involving the neonatal handling paradigm further support this connection. Neonatal handling during the first two weeks of life permanently reduces the HPA response to stress in adulthood. This reduction in HPA activity is, in part, mediated by a handling-induced increase in forebrain glucocorticoid receptor gene expression (Smythe et al 1994). Adult rats that have been handled early on in life have changes in both hippocampal and cortical GR and in hypothalamic CRH. In adulthood, these animals display increased hippocampal GR levels, decreased CRH in the PVN and enhanced negative feedback, which results in decreased HPA responsivity to stress (Meaney et al 1996). Interestingly, it has also been demonstrated that neonatal handling increases hippocampal serotonin levels and turnover (Mitchell et al 1990, Smythe et al 1994). Following this finding, the Meaney group showed that serotonin, acting by activating 5-HT_7 receptors, is involved in mediating the permanent upregulation of GR following neonatal handling (Meaney et al 2000). Furthermore, it has been reported that serotonin regulates hippocampal glucocorticoid receptor expression via the 5-HT_7 receptor in hippocampal cell cultures (Laplante et al 2002). For an excellent review on fetal programming of the HPA axis and serotonergic involvement see (Andrews & Matthews 2004) (Figure 10).

It is also possible that serotonin plays a role in programming of the HPA axis in animals prenatally exposed to ethanol. We have reported increased hippocampal 5-HT_{1A} mRNA levels in PAE compared to PF and C females in diestrus. This increase could be a compensatory mechanism due to the decrease in numbers of 5-HT neurons in adult PAE animals. Our recent unpublished data indicate that adult PAE ovariectomized females have a decrease of approximately 35% in the number of serotonin-immunoreactive (5HT-ir) neurons in the dorsal raphe nucleus of the brainstem (Sliwowska JH. et al., in preparation).This is a new and interesting finding, as it is the first example of alterations in the number of 5-HT-ir neurons in the brainstem of adult femalerats following PAE. This finding is in agreement with data from the Zhou laboratory showing that prenatal ethanol exposure results in fewer 5-HT-ir neurons in the dorsal raphe of male mice (Sari & Zhou 2004). Importantly, prenatal administration of 5-HT_{1A} agonists to pregnant dams has been shown to ameliorate some of the serotonergic deficits resulting from prenatal ethanol exposure in the offspring (Tajuddin & Druse 1993, Tajuddin & Druse 2001). Future studies in our laboratory will go on to explore a possible role for the hippocampal 5-HT_7 receptor in regulation of the HPA axis in PAE animals.

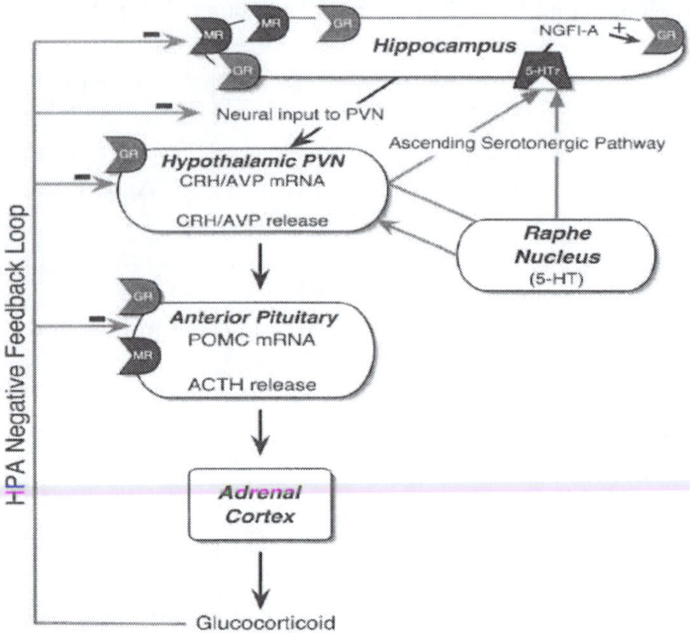

Figure 10. The fetal hypothalamic–pituitary–adrenal axis is controlled by positive drive (indicated by black arrows) and negative feedback (indicated by red arrows). The latter involves activation of glucocorticoid (GR) and mineralocorticoid (MR) receptors at various loci in the brain. At the level of the hippocampus, negative feedback activation of MR and GR by circulating glucocorticoids affects neural input to the PVN, where corticotrophin releasing hormone (CRH) and vasopressin (AVP) are produced. These two hormones stimulate proopiomelanocortin (POMC) mRNA transcription and increased adrenocorticotrophin (ACTH) release from the anterior pituitary, which, along with the PVN, is subject to negative feedback inhibition. Once released into peripheral circulation, ACTH stimulates the production and secretion of glucocorticoidsfrom the adrenal cortex, increasing the negative feedback signal. The HPA axis bi-directionally interacts with the serotonergic system. Ascending serotonergic neuronal pathways (indicated by green arrows), while originating in the raphe nucleus of the midbrain, project directly to the hypothalamus and the hippocampus, or innervate the hippocampus through intermediary relays (such as in the hypothalamus; reviewed in detail by Lowry, 2002). Activation of the hippocampal 5-HT_7 receptor, via increased activity of the transcription factor, NGFI-A, has been shown to increase fetal hippocampal GR expression (Meaney et al., 2000; Laplante et al., 2002). (Source: Reprinted and modified from Andrews MH. & Mathews SG. (2004) with permission from Taylor & Francis).

In summary, resetting of HPA activity by early environmental events could be a mechanism by which early life experiences are linked with long-term health. Thus, changes in basal CORT levels, shifts in the hippocampal

MR/GR balance and alterations in the 5-HT_{1A} receptor mRNA observed in our model of PAE could have important clinical implications. This could lead to an increased understanding of the secondary disabilities associated with prenatal alcohol exposure, such as the increased incidence of depression in children with FASD (see section twelve, chapter three).

The hippocampus is not only a unique region in which interactions between the serotonergic system and the HPA axis occur, but also a brain structure in which adult neurogenesis takes place and the effects of PAE on this process of hippocampal neurogenesis will be the focus of the next chapter.

10. Hippocampal Neurogenesis and Prenatal Alcohol Exposure

For over 100 years, a central dogma of neuroscience has been that, in the adult human, the loss of neurons is irreversible, as dying neurons cannot be replaced. In the early 1960's, Joseph Altman performed several studies using tritiatedthymidine (^{3}H-thymidine) autoradiography and showed the new neurons are present postnatally in rats in the neocortex, dentate gyrus and olfactory bulbs; however, these findings were neglected for quite some time. Fifteen years after Altman's initial findings, Kaplan showed autoradiographic and ultrastructural evidence for the existence of new neurons in the adult rat brain (Kaplan & Hinds 1977). Again, however, these findings did not receive much initial attention. Beginning around the 1990's, with development of the BrdU (5-bromo-3'-deoxyuridine) technique, additional proof of adult neurogenes is began to emerge. Studies performed by Gage and colleagues found that new neurons are generated in the dentate gyrus and the subventricular zone in adult humans /for a review on the history of adult neurogenesis see (Gross 2000)/.

In the rodent brain, new neurons are generated throughout life from a population of continuously dividing progenitor cells in the subgranular zone of the dentate gyrus and these neurons then migrate into the granule cell layer of the hippocampus, differentiate, extend axons and express neuronal marker proteins /for a review see (Eriksson et al 1998; Christie &Cameron 2006)/ (Figure11).

to an enriched environment. This later finding suggests that the neurogenic response to enrichment is altered with PAE (Choi et al 2005).

As the modulation of adult hippocampal neurogenesis by stress in PAE animals has yet to be examined, we have recently conducted studies to address this issue (Sliwowska et al. in press). We have investigated the effects of prenatal ethanol exposure and repeated stress in adulthood on both cell proliferation and cell survival in the hippocampus of adult male rats. We hypothesized that, in accordance with previous data from rat models, PAE would suppress basal levels of adult hippocampal neurogenesis. Furthermore, we hypothesized that stress, acting on a sensitized HPA axis, would have greater adverse effects on adult hippocampal neurogenesis in PAE compared to control animals. Indeed, we have found that under non-stressed conditions, PAE has a small but statistically significant suppressive effect on the level of hippocampal neurogenesis. Interestingly, repeated restraint stress reduces cell survival in C and PF, but not PAE rats. Based on the aforementioned examples, it seems that animals prenatally exposed to ethanol, when studied in adulthood, have impaired responses to environmental challenges, compared to controls. This is an interesting finding that is also seen in the context of aging, as studies in this area indicate that one of the clear signs of aging is an inappropriate response to environmental challenges. Thus, it is possible that PAE animals may age at a faster rate compared to controls. Noteably, animals prenatally exposed to ethanol, compare to controls, show earlier signs of reproductive system aging, as indicated by the loss of reproductive function (Li et al 1997; McGivern et al 1992; McGivern & Yellow 1992; Wilson & Handa 1997). Our unpublished data also indicate that PAE animals show delays in the onset of puberty (Sliwowska et al., in preparation). Thus, from this data, it is concluded that the reproductive window is decreased by prenatal ethanol exposure. It would be of interest to conduct further studies exploring aging at the level of the brain and in particular, the hippocampus and the hypothalamus, in order to begin to reveal the neuronal mechanisms associated with premature aging in PAE animals.

In contrast to our findings on cell survival under the stressed condition, there were no significant differences among prenatal groups in cell proliferation or dentate gyrus volume under either stressed or non-stressed conditions. Our finding of reduced hippocampal neurogenesis in PAE males under basal conditions is consistent with previous studies in rats, which have reported reductions in both cell proliferation and cell survival or reduced numbers of mature neurons in the dentate gyrus following prenatal ethanol exposure (Redila et al 2006). In contrast, a study in mice found no significant differences between PAE and control males in basal levels of adult hippocampal neurogenesis (Choi et al 2005). Methodological differences, including age, handling conditions, the species used and alcohol and BrdU administration paradigms may all influence the effects of PAE on cell proliferation and/or survival and these factors need to be considered when comparing results between studies /see (Sliwowska et al in press) for a discussion of these factors/. Interestingly, Mirescu and collaborators (Mirescu et al 2004), using an adult rat model of early maternal separation, also found impaired neurogenesis in early life and no effect on adult neurogenesis when animals were exposed to stress during adulthood. Early adverse experiences, such as prenatal and early postnatal stress, are associated with persistent changes in the HPA axis. Thus, these findings suggest that neurogenesis is inhibited in animals exposed to early life stressors because they either exhibit higher than normal levels of glucocorticoids or are hypersensitive to normal levels of these hormones. In agreement with this suggestion, lowering glucocorticoid levels below control values (by adrenalectomy) followed by low-dose corticosterone replacement restores the levels of cell proliferation in the DG of maternally separated animals to control levels (Mirescu et al 2004). It is also possible that corticosterone is responsible for the observed alterations in neurogenesis in our model. However, as mentioned earlier, in adulthood, PAE males usually do not have increased basal (non-stressed) corticosterone levels. Thus, hypersensitivity to normal levels of glucocorticoids could be proposed as a possible mechanism resulting in impaired neurogenesis in adult animals prenatally exposed to ethanol; however, further experiments are needed in order to substantiate this hypothesis.

Based on our findings, we propose that PAE impairs hippocampal neurogenesis and modulates regulation of adult neurogenesis in the DG following environmental challenges such as stress. We speculate that the failure of PAE males to mount an appropriate (i.e., suppressive) neurogenic response to stressors implies reduced plasticity, which could negatively impact hippocampal structure and function.

The female brain responds to steroid hormones differently than the male brain and adult the neurogenesis is differentially regulated in both sexes by gonadal and stress hormones /see reviews (Galea 2008; Galea et al. 2008)/. Thus, to expand further current experiments we are now examining the relationships between prenatal ethanol exposure, stress and hippocampal neurogenesis in female rats (Uban et al., in preparation). Taken together, we expect that these studies will provide us with a better understanding as to the role of PAE and stress on adult neurogenesisin both male and female rats.

11. Mechanisms of Action of Alcohol on the Hippocampus

Based on the above analysis, it is obvious that the hippocampus is sensitive to the teratogenic effects of prenatal alcohol exposure. The question that remains, however, concerns alcohol's mechanism of action on the hippocampus. The following chapter will review studies focusing on the changes in the hippocampus of animals prenatally exposed to ethanol.

A hallmark of FAS is microcephaly, which can result from either a reduction in: 1) the number of cells (neurons and/or glia), and/or 2) the volume of the neuropil, i.e., the amount of cellular processes (axons, dendrites and glial processes) (Miller 1996) and many investigators have studied this phenomenon. In the rat, neurons involved in hippocampal formation are generated from gestational day 15 into adulthood and PAE affects hippocampal cell numbers (Miller 1995). Miller and colleagues have shown that the total DNA and protein content of the hippocampus is lower in animals exposed to ethanol *in utero* compared to controls (Miller 1996). Additionally, PAE animals have fewer neurons in the pyramidal cell layer of CA1 and the granular cell layer of the DG compared to their control counterparts and they also display alterations in the distribution of mossy fibers in the hippocampal formation (Miller 1995; West et al 1981).

At this point, it is also important to note that, during development of the human brain, there are periods of rapid brain growth, which are recognized as being key developmental events. In the human, rapid brain growth begins at the end of the second trimester of gestation, reaching a peak at birth and gradually tapers off during the first few years of life (Dobbing & Sands 1979). In contrast, in the rat, these periods occur postnatally, starting at around postnatal day 4 (PND 4), with a peak of brain growth on PNDs 10-12, and with a subsequent decline occurring over the next two to three weeks. It is also important to keep in mind that the brain growth spurt is generally considered to be a very vulnerable period of brain development (Dobbing & Sands 1979, West et al 1987). In this context, the timing and duration of ethanol exposure, peak blood alcohol concentration and route of ethanol administration are all important variables to be considered when interpreting the results from animal studies of ethanol exposure (see section one, chapter three). Moreover, different investigators use different methods for estimating cell numbers. According to Coggeshall and colleagues (Coggeshall & Lekan 1996), the best currently available, unbiased serological method is the optical dissector procedure. Studies by West and colleagues, using the paradigm of third-trimester equivalent ethanol exposure, have reported reduced numbers of cells in the CA4 region and an increase in the number of cells in the DG but no change in cell numbers in the CA1 or CA3 regions (West et al 1986). However, in a study involving young rats (10 days old) prenatally exposed to ethanol (third trimester equivalent), a reduction in the number of pyramidal neurons in the CA1 region was reported. This same deficit was also found in 90 day old rats in a model of embryonic alcohol exposure (ethanol was administered from embryonic days 6 to 21). In a binge-like model of ethanol delivery during the first and second trimester-equivalents, Maier and West did not find changes in the number of CA1, CA3 and DG cells compared to controls (Maier & West 2001). Based on the above examples, it is obvious that more studies are needed focusing on the teratogenic effect of alcohol on the hippocampus.

Regardless of alcohol's mechanism of action on the hippocampus, the long-term devastating consequences of alcohol on this brain structure are undeniable. The next chapter will bring the data together and propose some of the potential long-term implications of prenatal alcohol exposure.

12. Prenatal Stress, Prenatal Alcohol Exposure and Dysregulationof the HPA Axis and the Hippocampus: Implications for the Neurobiology of Depression

As previously mentioned, both children and adults with FAS experience higher rates of mental disorders, including depression and anxiety, compared to the normal population (Famy et al 1998, O'Connor & Paley 2006, Streissguth et al 1996). Altered function of the HPA and 5-HT systems are known to be critical factors involved in the etiology of depression (Lopez et al 1998, Nestler et al 2002, Pryce et al 2005). These systems are also altered in adults and children prenatally exposed to alcohol (see chapter three, sections eight and nine). Moreover, the hippocampus, a region in which MR, GR, 5-HT_{1A} and 5-HT_7 receptors are particularly abundant, represents a unique anatomical environment in which to study the interplay between the serotonergic and HPA systems (Lopez et al 1998). Additionally, as mentioned in chapter three, section three, several cases of decreased hippocampal volume have been reported in children with FASD. A recent review of the available data on hippocampal volume in depressed patients has also shown a reduction in hippocampal volume following the onset of major depression /for a review see (McKinnon et al 2009)/. Finally, the hippocampus is a highly stress-sensitive brain region and FASD and depression are highly stress-sensitive illnesses (Kessler 1997, Weinberg et al 2008).

In light of the above-mentioned evidence, it is very important to study the long-term effects of prenatal ethanol exposure and its role in fetal programming and later life vulnerability to stress and depression. Indeed, in our rat model of prenatal ethanol exposure, offspring in adulthood share the hormonal changes characteristic of depression: 1) increased HPA drive; 2) deficits in HPA feedback regulation, which are manifested by increased corticosterone levels, earlier escape from dexamethasone suppression, increased ACTH responsiveness to dexamethasone and CRH (challenge tests used to assess depression) (Holsboer 2000); 3) hippocampal MR/GR imbalances; and 4) alterations in the serotonergic system (e.g. decreased numbers of 5-HT-ir neurons and alterations in 5-HT_{1A} receptor mRNA levels), which together could disrupt the interactions between the HPA and the 5-HT systems and in turn, underlie, at least in part, the increased vulnerability to depression seen in children and adults with FASD /see reviews: (Sliwowska et al 2006, Weinberg et al 2008)/ (Figure12).

Findings obtained using our model of prenatal ethanol exposure are relevant to other rodent studies as well as to *post-mortem* findings in humans. For example, studies by Lopez and colleagues (Lopez et al 1998) reveal that rats subjected to chronic, unpredictable stress (experimental paradigm used in animal models of depression-like behaviours, mimicking chronic, unpredictable stress in humans) exhibit elevations in basal plasma CORT, decreases in 5-HT_{1A} mRNA in the hippocampus, decreases in hippocampal MR mRNA levels and alterations in the MR/GR ratio in adulthood. Importantly, these changes can be reversed through antidepressant treatment with serotonin reuptake inhibitors (imipramine or desipramine) and these compounds are acting possibly by decreasing the stress-induced corticosteroid elevations. Consistent with theses animal studies, suicide victims with a history of major depression tend to have lower MR mRNA levels, decreased 5-HT_{1A} and no change in GR mRNA levels in the hippocampus suggesting a possible mechanism by which stress can trigger and/or maintain depressive episodes (Lopez et al 1998).

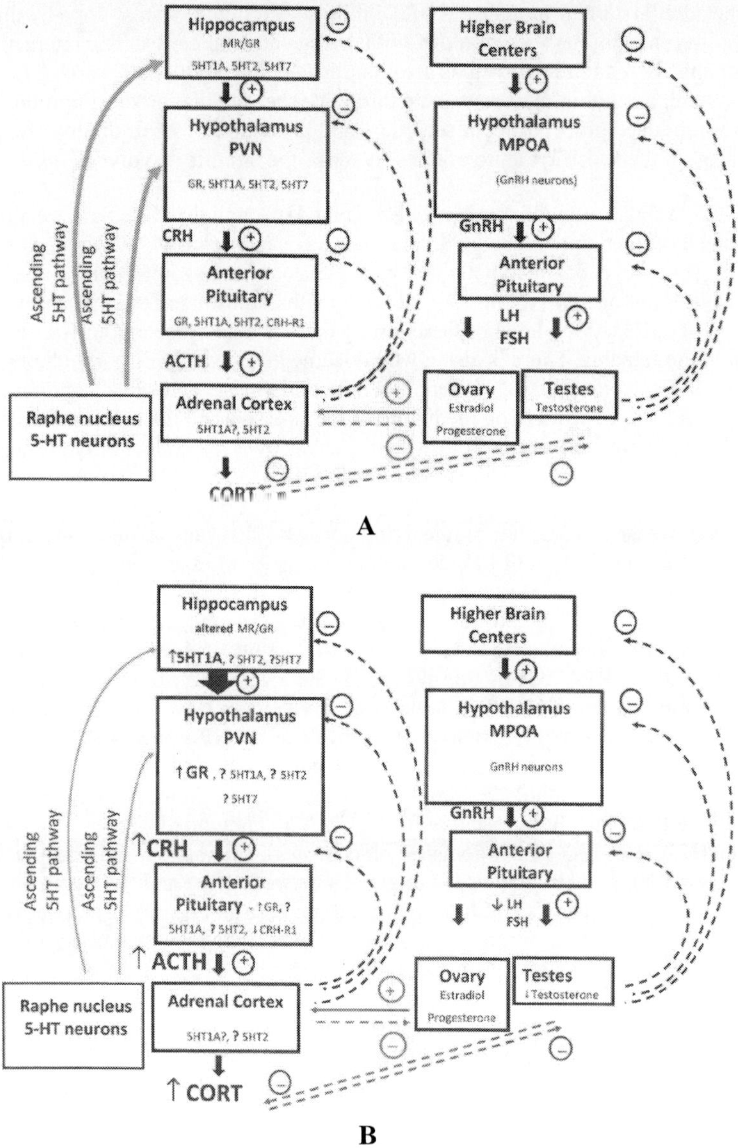

Figure 12. Model of the interactions among the HPA axis,the HPG axis and the 5-HT system in normal (A) and in PAE animals (B). (A) In normal animals there is a cascade of hormones secreted by the HPA and the HPG axis controlled by positive and negative feedback. There are bidirectional and sex specific interactions between the HPA and the HPG axis. In general stress inhibits reproductive functions and in turn, the gonadal steroids modulate HPA activity at all levels of the axis. In females, CORT inhibits secretion of estradiol by the ovaries and estradiol stimulates CORT secretion

from the adrenal cortex. In males, CORT inhibits secretion of testosterone by the testis and testosterone inhibits secretion of CORT by the adrenal cortex. The interactions between the HPA and the HPG axis are complicated and additionally modulated by the 5-HT system. Serotonin may contribute through either facilitation or inhibition of basal and stress-induced glucocorticoid secretion, and the action of serotonin may be dependent on the specific nature of the stressor or the circuitry involved.

(B) In PAE animals, the interactions between the HPA and the HPG axis are altered. At the level of the hippocampus, PAE animals have an altered MR/GR receptor balance. At the level of the hypothalamus, there is an increase in GR and an increase in stimulatory input or drive to the PVN of the hypothalamus manifested as an increased secretion of CRH. At the level of the pituitary there is a decrease in CRH-R1 in males but not in the females. There is also a well documented sexually dimorphic increase in secretion of CORT and/or ACTH reported both under basal and stress conditions or under stress only, dependent on the nature of the stressor, and the time course and hormonal endpoints measured. Following the stress of chronic alcohol exposure in adulthood, PAE males show increased pituitary GR, whereas PAE females show decreased pituitary GR levels. The HPG axis is also altered in PAE animals such that there is a decrease in secretion of lutenizing hormone (LH) and testosterone in males and a decrease in secretion of LH, delayed sexual maturation and onset of follicle-stimulating hormone (FSH) secretion in females. There are also changes in sensitivity to sex steroids (estradiol and testosterone).The 5-HT system is also altered in PAE animals. There is a decrease in the ascending 5-HTpathways leading to altered modulation of the HPA axis by this system. At the levels of the hippocampus we have reported an increase in 5-HT1A in females during diestrus (low estradiol level). The modulatoryrole of the 5-HT system at other levels of the HPA axis in PAE animals as well as sexually dimorphic differences in these interactions in PAE animals is currently not well understood.Symbols: + stimulation; - inhibition;solid black lines - positive feedback; dotted black lines negative feedback; ?– unknown;red arrows – interactions between HPA and HPG axis in females; blue arrows – interactions between HPA and HPG axis in males; green arrows – interactions between HPA and 5HT systems. Thicker and thinner arrows and fonts represent increase and decrease, respectively. HPA – the hypothalamic-pituitary-adrenal axis; HPG – the hypothalamic-pituitary-gonadal axis; 5-HT-serotonergic system; PAE – prenatal ethanol exposure; PF – pair-fed; C – control.

In light of the relationship between adverse early life events and depression in adulthood (Gutman & Nemeroff 2003), it is proposed that prenatal ethanol exposure can be viewed as an early life stressor that sensitizes or primes the neurobiological stress systems. Thus,individuals exposed to alcohol *in utero* are hyperactive in their response to subsequent, even mild, stressful life events and ultimately have increased vulnerability to depression and other stress-related disorders. In the context of the stress-diathesis model, it is proposed that fetal programming of the HPA axis by PAE alters neuroadaptive mechanisms that mediate the stress response, thus sensitizing the organism to stressors encountered later in life and mediating, at least partly, the increased vulnerability to depression/anxiety disorders. The hippocampus, as a regulatory structure of the HPA axis, is particularly vulnerable to the teratogenic effects of alcohol and this critical brain region needs to be further studied in order to better understand the long-term effects of prenatal ethanol exposure. A more in depth grasp of the anatomical and functional abnormalities of this brain structure, caused by alcohol, should help us to design therapeutic tools, which could be used to treat individuals experiencing the devastating effects of prenatal alcohol exposure.

Chapter IV

Can We Prevent or Reverse the Effects of Prenatal Alcohol Exposure on the Hippocampus? Intervention, Prevention and Implication

Prior to delving into a discussion of prevention and intervention strategies for FASD, it is important to consider the factors that contribute to the variable profiles of brain damage associated with FASD. These include: maternal factors, e.g. time, frequency and duration of alcohol abuse during pregnancy; socioeconomic status, e.g., poverty, smoking or other drug use, nutritional deficiencies, poor prenatal care or support, disadvantaged postnatal environments, and genetic factors, e.g.ADH2*3 alleles which code for a more efficient alcohol dehydrogenase enzyme, decreasing the risk of FAS in the infant as well as maternal and fetal genotype which can impact the susceptibility to alcohol teratogenesis under conditions of comparable alcohol exposure /for details, see the review (Goodlett et al 2005)/.

As previously discussed (chapter three, section eleven), it has been well established that prenatal alcohol exposure damages the brain, including the hippocampus, and that this occurs via multiple mechanisms. Alcohol can interact with or functionally alter many target molecules, including receptors and ion channels, cell signaling proteins, metabolic enzymes and lipids /for a review see (Goodlett et al 2005)/. Despite the complexity of the neurological or physiological effects of alcohol, attempts are being made to identify candidate mechanisms of action giving rise to brain damage in FASD. Understanding the mechanism(s) of alcohol's action is crucial for the development of possible interventions, which will be discussed below. Interventions can be implemented at the pharmacological as well the behavioral level in order to lessen the burden of FASD. Intervention strategies have been extensively reviewed by Goodlett and colleagues /see (Goodlett & Horn 2001, Goodlett et al 2005)/. Here, the focus is only on several key candidate mechanisms as well as the most pertinent pharmacological interventions and therapeutic agents that may alleviate some of the damage to the hippocampus caused by PAE.

1. Pharmacological Interventions

1.1. Disruption of Serotonergic Neural Development: Treatment with 5-HT_{1A} Agonists and the Role of Estradiol

The effect of prenatal ethanol exposure on the serotonergic system has received special attention due to the role of 5-HT,which acts as a neurotropic factor (Azmitia 2002). The 5-HT system is also one of the earliest transmitter systems to develop during ontogeny and it is hypothesized that serotonin is an important signaling chemical involved in neuronal development as well as overall maturation of the central nervous system (Whitaker-Azmitia et al 1996). Thus, early insult to the 5HT neurons may affect not only the development of this system but also that of other neurotransmitter networks. There exists a large body of evidence suggesting that animals prenatally exposed to ethanol display compromised development of 5-HT neurons. Specific abnormalities include deficiencies in serotonin and its metabolites, reduced cortical 5-HT reuptake sites, decreases in the number of 5-HT neurons, decreased serotonergic innervations and deficits in the concentration of 5-HT_{1A} receptors (Druse et al 1991, Rathbun & Druse 1985, Sari & Zhou 2004, Sliwowska et al 2008, Zhou et al 2005, Zhou et al 2001). PAE animals also have behavioral abnormalities consistent with altered 5-HT functioning including anxiety and aggression (Hofmann et al 2007, Hofmann et al 2005, Hofmann et al 2002) and it is thorough these animal models that possible prevention strategies are being examined. It has been hypothesized that 5-HT_{1A} agonists act as neuroprotective agents by reducing apoptosis (a form of programmed cell death or "cell suicide") in 5-HT as well as other types of neurons. In fact, treatment with the 5-HT_{1A} agonists buspirone and ipsapirone prevent the development of deficits in the serotonergic system which are commonly associated with prenatal ethanol exposure (Druse et al 2004, Eriksen & Druse 2001, Kim & Druse 1996, Tajuddin & Druse 1993). Thus, the aforementioned studies suggest that treatment with 5-HT_{1A} agonists is a promising treatment strategy that could act as a potential pharmacotherapeutic intervention in the case of heavy, ongoing maternal drinking, which places the offspring at risk for FASD (Goodlett et al 2005).This is also important in the context of alcohol's effects on the hippocampus, since this region is innervated by 5-HT neurons and contains serotonin receptors. Moreover, we have found that hippocampal 5-HT_{1A} receptor mRNA levels are increased during the diestrus stage of the estrus cycle in adult females prenatally exposed to ethanol (Sliwowska et al 2008). Our recent unpublished data (Sliwowska et al. in preparation) also show that PAE females, when ovariectomized as adults, have a decrease in the number of serotonergic neurons in the dorsal raphe. Interestingly, this decrease is prevented by a two week replacement with physiological levels of estradiol. Thus, in addition to 5-HT_{1A} agonists, estradiol (at least in case of females and in our paradigm) could potentially protect the 5-HT system against the damaging effects of PAE. However, future studies are required to explore this possibility. Besides 5-HT_{1A} receptors, based on the importance of hippocampal 5-HT_7 receptors in fetal programming (see chapter three, section six,), another promising new area of research in the field of FASD intervention could include targeting this serotonin receptor subtype.

1.2. Treatment with Activity-Dependent Neuroprotective Peptides

Alcohol impairs growth of the central nervous system and induces neurodegeneration through cellular apoptosis. Thus, another promising treatment strategy in the field of FASD involves peptides that have been shown to play a role in neuroprotection. Among these peptides are: 1) Activity-dependent neuroprotective protein (ADNP); 2) Activity-dependent neuroprotective factor (ADNF); 3) NAP (a peptide with the sequence NAPVSIPQ, derived from ADNP); 4) SAL or ADNF-9 (a peptide with the sequence SALLRSIPA derived from ADNF) /for a review see (Sari & Gozes 2006)/.

Importantly, *in vitro* studies have shown that amino acid fragment of ADNF (ADNF-9) protects cultured rat hippocampal neurons from oxidative stress and neuronal apoptosis (Glazner et al 1999). In addition, pretreatment with NAP alone or in combination with NAP and SAL has been found to prevent fetal death and other abnormalities induced by prenatal alcohol exposure (Spong et al 2001). Of particular interest is a study performed by Vink and colleagues showing that male mice prenatally exposed to ethanol display learning deficits in the Morris water maze in adulthood, effects which can be prevented by pretreating with NAP and ADNF-9 (Vink et al 2005). Administration of SAL also antagonizes the effects of alcohol on the body as well as brain weight and growth and the development of various brain structural deficits, including hippocampal alterations in a mouse model of FAS (Zhou et al 2004).

Thus, these studies involving treatment with Activity-dependent neuroprotective peptides seem to suggest that this may be a promising new area of research in the field of FASD intervention. However, prior to being able to apply ADNP's as a therapeutic agent in the treatment of FASD in human patients, a more detailed understanding of the intracellular targets and downstream mechanism of action of these peptides is required.

1.3. Oxidative Stress and Free Radical Damage: Prevention with Antioxidant Supplements

Oxidative stress, the imbalance between the formation and degradation of reactive oxygen species (ROS), has been implicated as playing a role in ethanol-induced toxicity in the brain (Bailey et al 1999, Kurose et al 1997, Montoliu et al 1994). The alcohol-induced formation of excess levels of ROS can result in cell death by interfering with mitochondrial functioning (mitochondria being organelles that generate the majority of the cell's energy) (Goodlett & Horn 2001). Antioxidant supplementation (e.g. Vitamin C, Vitamin E, b-carotene) has been shown to prevent some of the ethanol-induced damage or pathogenesis in animal models of PAE (Goodlett et al 2005). Importantly, Vitamin E and b-carotene supplementation prevents ethanol-induced cell loss in embryonic rat hippocampal cultures (Mitchell et al 1999). Thus, supplementation with antioxidants has been suggested as a potential treatment to prevent ethanol toxicity during development.

2. Behavioral Interventions

In addition to pharmacological interventions, behavioral therapies are a potential avenue being explored in the treatment of FASD. However, it is important to note that pharmacological and behavioral approaches are not exclusive and should, ideally, be applied in combination. Despite considerable data published on cognitive and behavioral disabilities in children with FASD, relatively little information is available on behavioral interventions for alcohol-affected children. A PubMed search of the terms "behavioral interventions and FAS" revealed only 37 papers dedicated to this topic and replacing the term FASD with FAS further decreased the result to only 17 relevant papers. Out of these 17 papers, only four were published in last year (2009) (Coles et al 2009, Kodituwakku 2009, Olson et al 2009, Peadon et al 2009). Importantly, as emphasized by Peadon and colleagues in their systematic review of interventions for children with FASD, many of these studies suffer from methodological weaknesses, including small sample sizes, inadequate study design and a lack of short term follow-up (Peadon et al 2009).

The limited progress in the development of evidence-based interventions for alcohol-affected children is puzzling given that successful animal models of interventions in FASD have been well established /e.g. (Berman & Hannigan 2000, Berman et al 1996, Hannigan et al 1993, Klintsova et al 1998, Wainwright et al 1993)/.

This section will focus on animal studies and present examples, which may be useful in the development of strategies to ameliorate the effects of prenatal alcohol exposure on hippocampal-dependent behaviours in humans. Firstly, it is important to review the elegant studies by Berman and Hannigan summarizing findings of changes in hippocampal-related tasks following prenatal ethanol exposure (Berman & Hannigan 2000). These researchers have reported that PAE animals are impaired in many spatial learning and memory tasks that rely on the hippocampus, including the T-maze, the Morris water maze, and the radial arm maze. They have also found that these deficits tend to be greater in both younger animals and following high doses of alcohol (as measured by higher peak blood alcohol concentrations - BACs). Based on the pattern of spatial learning and memory deficits, it is suggested that direct hippocampal damage has occurred. This finding supports the hypothesis that PAE interferes with normal development and functioning of the hippocampus (Riley et al 1986). However, it remains to be seen if these alcohol-related changes are in fact reversible and if performance could be improved with an early behavioral intervention approach.

2.2. Enriched or Complex Environments

Rearing animals in enriched or complex environments reliably stimulates central nervous system development, facilitating recovery of function and enhancing behavioral performance (Kolb et al 1998, Rosenzweig 1996, Weiler et al 1995). Thus, this strategy seems promising and applicable as an intervention potentially capable of reversing or decreasing the neurological damage caused by ethanol. Several investigators have used this technique and report that rearing PAE animals (rats and mice) in an enriched environment can improve behavioral performance in learning, memory and motor tasks (Berman et al 1996, Hannigan et al 1993, Klintsova et al 1998, Wainwright et al 1993). However, other studies have found that these enriched environments to do not affect the performance of PAE mice and rats on several behavioral tasks (Choi et al 2005, Opitz et al 1997, Osborne et al 1980). The discrepancy in results suggests that the effects of enrichment may depend on other factors such as the dose and/or periods of alcohol exposure, the species in question, the severity of fetal alcohol effects, the age at which enrichment is applied and the specific behavioral task being assessed. Interestingly, studies by Berman and colleagues (Berman et al 1996) also show that, following prenatal ethanol exposure in rats, environmental enrichment does not increase spine density, suggesting decreased neural plasticity in adulthood in PAE animals.Thus, a reduction in the neuroanatomical plasticity of the hippocampus may be associated with the cognitive impairments characteristic of FASD (Berman et al 1996).

2.3. Voluntary Exercise: Running

Another promising behavioral intervention is the implementation of increased physical activity, which is modeled in animal studies by voluntary running in wheels. Importantly, animals reared in enriched environments (see above) as well as those partaking in running show increased neurogenesis in the dentate gyrus (van Praag 2008, van Praag et al 1999a, van Praag et al 1999b). Additionally, in humans and rodents, physical activity has also been shown to give rise to enhanced cognition (Rogers et al 1990, Suominen-Troyer et al 1986, van Praag et al 1999a, Winter et al 2007). The above-mentioned advantages of physical activity have led to the hypothesis that the beneficial effects of running onmood and cognition may be mediated, at least in part, by enhanced hippocampal neurogenesis. Consequently, it has been shown that running improves Morris water maze performance, increases the numbers of new neurons and enhances dentate gyrus LTP in mice (van Praag et al 1999a, van Praag et al 1999b).

Studies by the Christie group have explored the potential role of running in the rat model of prenatal ethanol exposure. They have shown that rats prenatally exposed to ethanol have decreased cell proliferation and survival in the dentate gyrus of the hippocampus as adults. Importantly, they have also reported that in adulthood, PAE male rats engaged in voluntary exercise, show a significant increase in cell proliferation and neurogenesis (Redila et al 2006). Despite the increase in neurogenesis seen in PAE rats, exercise does not raise the number of new neurons born to the level achieved in control rat runners. Thus, it seems that physical activity, at least in the context of voluntary running, enhances hippocampal neurogenesis in PAE adult rats. However, prenatal ethanol exposure also seems to impair adult neurogenic responses such that the PAE animals do not benefit from running to the same degree as control animals. Additional studies by Christie and colleagues show that exposure to ethanol *in utero* impairs spatial memory and LTP in male rats, a finding that is attenuated by voluntary exercise (Christie et al 2005). Together, the above-mentioned benefits of voluntary exercise suggest that this may be of therapeutic relevance in the treatment of individuals with FASD.

3. Implications for Human FASD

In this section, the implications of animal studies on the human condition of FASD are discussed and strategies that may prove beneficial in the field of prevention and intervention are outlined.

FASD can be prevented either by abstinence from alcohol during pregnancy or by preventing reproduction in alcohol-abusing women of childbearing age. In spite of substantial effort, these prevention approaches have not proven successful and as a result, interventions with the goal of limiting the health-related burden of prenatal ethanol exposure are needed /see (Goodlett et al 2005)/. One of the approaches proposed by Goodlett and colleagues is to implement specific pharmacotherapeutic interventions during pregnancy and make them available to at-risk populations, where the incidence of FASD is high (Goodlett et al 2005). Based on the above discussion these interventions may include antioxidant supplements as well as treatment with 5-HT agonists and Activity-dependent neuroprotective peptides. The other approach, in combination with pharmacological agents, is behavioral intervention (e.g. environmental enrichment), which in humans could be translated as social support. Another emerging behavioral intervention, based on the animal studies discussed above, is increased physical activity. All of the above mentioned strategies either directly or indirectly work on enhancing hippocampal function, as this structure is impaired in animal models of PAE and in humans prenatally exposed to alcohol.

Chapter V

General Conclusion

The aim of this book was to provide evidence in support of the hypothesis that prenatal alcohol exposure interferes with the normal development and function of the hippocampus. I hope that readers were able to find, in the pages of this book, a wide array of anatomical, histological, physiological and behavioral support of this hypothesis. I also hope that readers will start to appreciate that emerging therapeutic strategies provide us with hope for improving the lives of individuals experiencing the devastating effects of prenatal alcohol exposure.

References

Abel EL. 1997. Was the fetal alcohol syndrome recognized in the ancient Near East? *Alcohol Alcohol.* 32: 3-7

Abel EL. 1999. Was the fetal alcohol syndrome recognized by the Greeks and Romans? *Alcohol Alcohol.* 34: 868-72

Abel EL. 2001. Gin Lane: did Hogarth know about fetal alcohol syndrome? *Alcohol Alcohol.* 36: 131-4

Amaral DLP. 2007. Hippocampal neuroanatomy. In *The Hppocampus Book*, ed. MR Andersen P., Amaral D., Bliss T., O'Keefe J., pp. p. 37-114. New York: Oxford University Press

Andrews MH, Matthews SG. 2004. Programming of the hypothalamo-pituitary-adrenal axis: serotonergic involvement. *Stress.* 7: 15-27

Angevine JB, Jr. 1965. Time of neuron origin in the hippocampal region. An autoradiographic study in the mouse. *Exp. Neurol. Suppl*: Suppl 2:1-70

Archibald SL, Fennema-Notestine C, Gamst A, Riley EP, Mattson SN, Jernigan TL. 2001. Brain dysmorphology in individuals with severe prenatal alcohol exposure. *Dev. Med. Child Neurol.* 43: 148-54

Arnold SE, Trojanowski JQ. 1996. Human fetal hippocampal development: I. Cytoarchitecture, myeloarchitecture, and neuronal morphologic features. *J. Comp. Neurol.* 367: 274-92

Astley S. 2009. *MRI, MRS and fMRI study of children with FASD.* Presented at The 3rd International Conference on Fetal Alcohol Spectrum Disorder., Victoria, BC, Canada

Atkinson HC, Waddell BJ. 1997. Circadian variation in basal plasma corticosterone and adrenocorticotropin in the rat: sexual dimorphism and changes across the estrous cycle. *Endocrinology.* 138: 3842-8

Autti-Ramo I, Autti T, Korkman M, Kettunen S, Salonen O, Valanne L. 2002. MRI findings in children with school problems who had been exposed prenatally to alcohol. *Dev. Med. Child Neurol.* 44: 98-106

Avishai-Eliner S, Brunson KL, Sandman CA, Baram TZ. 2002. Stressed-out, or in (utero)? *Trends Neurosci.* 25:518-24

Azmitia EC. 2002. Cajal's hypotheses on neurobiones and neurotropic factor match properties of microtubules and S-100 beta. *Prog. Brain Res.* 136: 87-100

Bailey SM, Pietsch EC, Cunningham CC. 1999. Ethanol stimulates the production of reactive oxygen species at mitochondrial complexes I and III. *Free Radic. Biol. Med.* 27: 891-900

Bakker JM, van Bel F, Heijnen CJ. 2001. Neonatal glucocorticoids and the developing brain: short-term treatment with life-long consequences? *Trends Neurosci.* 24: 649-53

Barbazanges A, Piazza PV, Le Moal M, Maccari S. 1996. Maternal glucocorticoid secretion mediates long-term effects of prenatal stress. *J. Neurosci.* 16: 3943-9

Barker DJ, Osmond C, Golding J, Kuh D, Wadsworth ME. 1989. Growth in utero, blood pressure in childhood and adult life, and mortality from cardiovascular disease. *Bmj.* 298: 564-7

Barr HM, Bookstein FL, O'Malley KD, Connor PD, Huggins JE, Streissguth AP. 2006. Binge drinking during pregnancy as a predictor of psychiatric disorders on the Structured Clinical Interview for DSM-IV in young adult offspring. *Am. J. Psychiatry.* 163: 1061-5

Bayer SA. 1980. Development of the hippocampal region in the rat. I. Neurogenesis examined with 3H-thymidine autoradiography. *J. Comp. Neurol.* 190: 87-114

Benediktsson R, Calder AA, Edwards CR, Seckl JR. 1997. Placental 11 beta-hydroxysteroid dehydrogenase: a key regulator of fetal glucocorticoid exposure. *Clin. Endocrinol. (Oxf)* 46: 161-6

Berman RF, Hannigan JH. 2000. Effects of prenatal alcohol exposure on the hippocampus: spatial behavior, electrophysiology, and neuroanatomy. *Hippocampus.* 10: 94-110

Berman RF, Hannigan JH, Sperry MA, Zajac CS. 1996. Prenatal alcohol exposure and the effects of environmental enrichment on hippocampal dendritic spine density. *Alcohol.* 13: 209-16

Brown J, Cooper-Kuhn CM, Kempermann G, Van Praag H, Winkler J, et al. 2003. Enriched environment and physical activity stimulate hippocampal but not olfactory bulb neurogenesis. *Eur. J. Neurosci.* 17: 2042-6

Burgess LH, Handa RJ. 1992. Chronic estrogen-induced alterations in adrenocorticotropin and corticosterone secretion, and glucocorticoid receptor-mediated functions in female rats. *Endocrinology.* 131: 1261-9

Cadet R, Pradier P, Dalle M, Delost P. 1986. Effects of prenatal maternal stress on the pituitary adrenocortical reactivity in guinea-pig pups. *J. Dev. Physiol.* 8: 467-75

Cameron HA, Gould E. 1994. Adult neurogenesis is regulated by adrenal steroids in the dentate gyrus. *Neuroscience.* 61: 203-9

Cameron HA, McKay RD. 2001. Adult neurogenesis produces a large pool of new granule cells in the dentate gyrus. *J. Comp. Neurol.* 435: 406-17

Carey MP, Deterd CH, de Koning J, Helmerhorst F, de Kloet ER. 1995. The influence of ovarian steroids on hypothalamic-pituitary-adrenal regulation in the female rat. *J. Endocrinol.* 144: 311-21

Choi IY, Allan AM, Cunningham LA. 2005. Moderate fetal alcohol exposure impairs the neurogenic response to an enriched environment in adult mice. *Alcohol. Clin. Exp. Res.* 29: 2053-62

Christie BR, Cameron HA. 2006. Neurogenesis in adult hippocampus. *Hippocampus.* 16: 199-207

Christie BR, Swann SE, Fox CJ, Froc D, Lieblich SE, et al. 2005. Voluntary exercise rescues deficits in spatial memory and long-term potentiation in prenatal ethanol-exposed male rats. *Eur. J. Neurosci.* 21: 1719-26

Chrousos GP. 1995. The hypothalamic-pituitary-adrenal axis and immune-mediated inflammation. *N. Engl. J. Med.* 332: 1351-62

Coe CL, Kramer M, Czeh B, Gould E, Reeves AJ, et al. 2003. Prenatal stress diminishes neurogenesis in the dentate gyrus of juvenile rhesus monkeys. *Biol. Psychiatry.* 54: 1025-34

Coggeshall RE, Lekan HA. 1996. Methods for determining numbers of cells and synapses: a case for more uniform standards of review. *J. Comp. Neurol.* 364: 6-15

Coles CD, Kable JA, Taddeo E. 2009. Math performance and behavior problems in children affected by prenatal alcohol exposure: intervention and follow-up. *J. Dev. Behav. Pediatr.*30: 7-15

Conference. NCD. 1995. Effect of corticosteroids for fetal maturation and perinatal outcomes. In: *Am. J. Obstet. Gynecol.* 235-344

Corkin S, Amaral DG, Gonzalez RG, Johnson KA, Hyman BT. 1997. H. M.'s medial temporal lobe lesion: findings from magnetic resonance imaging. *J. Neurosci.* 17: 3964-79

Crews FT, Nixon K. 2003. Alcohol, neural stem cells, and adult neurogenesis. *Alcohol Res. Health.* 27: 197-204

Cudd TA. 2005. Animal model systems for the study of alcohol teratology. *Exp. Biol. Med. (Maywood)* 230: 389-93

Dallman MF. 2003. Stress by any other name .....? *Horm. Behav.* 43: 18-20; discussion 8-30

Davis VE. 1980. The fetus and alcohol. *Med. J. Aust.* 1: 558

de Kloet ER, Joels M, Holsboer F. 2005. Stress and the brain: from adaptation to disease. *Nat. Rev. Neurosci.* 6: 463-75

de Kloet ER, Reul JM, Sutanto W. 1990. Corticosteroids and the brain. *J. Steroid. Biochem. Mol. Biol.* 37: 387-94

De Kloet ER, Vreugdenhil E, Oitzl MS, Joels M. 1998. Brain corticosteroid receptor balance in health and disease. *Endocr. Rev.* 19: 269-301

Dean F, Matthews SG. 1999. Maternal dexamethasone treatment in late gestation alters glucocorticoid and mineralocorticoid receptor mRNA in the fetal guinea pig brain. *Brain Res.* 846: 253-9

Dobbing J, Sands J. 1979. Comparative aspects of the brain growth spurt. *Early Hum. Dev.* 3: 79-83

Druse MJ, Kuo A, Tajuddin N. 1991. Effects of in utero ethanol exposure on the developing serotonergic system. *Alcohol Clin. Exp. Res.* 15: 678-84

Druse MJ, Tajuddin NF, Gillespie RA, Dickson E, Atieh M, et al. 2004. The serotonin-1A agonist ipsapirone prevents ethanol-associated death of total rhombencephalic neurons and prevents the reduction of fetal serotonin neurons. *Brain Res. Dev. Brain Res.* 150: 79-88

Duman RS, Malberg J, Nakagawa S, D'Sa C. 2000. Neuronal plasticity and survival in mood disorders. *Biol. Psychiatry.* 48: 732-9

Eriksen JL, Druse MJ. 2001. Astrocyte-mediated trophic support of developing serotonin neurons: effects of ethanol, buspirone, and S100B. *Brain Res. Dev. Brain Res.* 131: 9-15

Eriksson PS, Perfilieva E, Bjork-Eriksson T, Alborn AM, Nordborg C, et al. 1998. Neurogenesis in the adult human hippocampus. *Nat. Med.* 4: 1313-7

Famy C, Streissguth AP, Unis AS. 1998. Mental illness in adults with fetal alcohol syndrome or fetal alcohol effects. *Am. J. Psychiatry.* 155: 552-4

Figueiredo HF, Dolgas CM, Herman JP. 2002. Stress activation of cortex and hippocampus is modulated by sex and stage of estrus. *Endocrinology.* 143: 2534-40

Frotscher M, Seress L. 2007. Morphological development of the hippocampus. In *The Hippocampus Book*, ed. MR Andersen P., Amaral D., Bliss T., O'Keefe J., pp. p.115-31. New York: Oxford University Press

Gallo PV, Weinberg J. 1981. Corticosterone rhythmicity in the rat: interactive effects of dietary restriction and schedule of feeding. *J. Nutr.* 111: 208-18

Gillies GE, Linton EA, Lowry PJ. 1982. Corticotropin releasing activity of the new CRF is potentiated several times by vasopressin. *Nature*. 299: 355-7

Glavas MM, Ellis L, Yu WK, Weinberg J. 2007. Effects of prenatal ethanol exposure on basal limbic-hypothalamic-pituitary-adrenal regulation: role of corticosterone. *Alcohol Clin. Exp. Res.* 31: 1598-610

Glazner GW, Boland A, Dresse AE, Brenneman DE, Gozes I, Mattson MP. 1999. Activity-dependent neurotrophic factor peptide (ADNF9) protects neurons against oxidative stress-induced death. *J. Neurochem.* 73: 2341-7

Galea LA. 2008. Gonadal hormone modulation of neurogenesis in the dentate gyrus of adult male and female rodents. *Brain Res Rev.* 57:332-41

Galea LA, Uban KA, Epp JR, Brummelte S, Barha CK, Wilson WL, Lieblich SE, Pawluski JL. 2008. Endocrine regulation of cognition and neuroplasticity: our pursuit to unveil the complex interaction between hormones, the brain, and behaviour. *Can J Exp Psychol.* 62:247-60.

Godfrey KM, Barker DJ. 2000. Fetal nutrition and adult disease. *Am. J. Clin. Nutr.* 71: 1344S-52S

Golgi C, Bentivoglio M, Swanson L. 2001. On the fine structure of the pes Hippocampi major (with plates XIII-XXIII). 1886. *Brain Res. Bull.* 54: 461-83

Goodlett CR, Horn KH. 2001. Mechanisms of alcohol-induced damage to the developing nervous system. *Alcohol Res. Health.* 25: 175-84

Goodlett CR, Horn KH, Zhou FC. 2005. Alcohol teratogenesis: mechanisms of damage and strategies for intervention. *Exp. Biol. Med. (Maywood)* 230: 394-406

Gould E. 2007. Structural plasticity. In *The Hippocampus Book*, ed. MR Andersen P., Amaral D., Bliss T., O'Keefe J., pp. p.332-5. New York: Oxford University Press

Gould E, Cameron HA, Daniels DC, Woolley CS, McEwen BS. 1992. Adrenal hormones suppress cell division in the adult rat dentate gyrus. *J. Neurosci.* 12: 3642-50

Gould E, Tanapat P, Hastings NB, Shors TJ. 1999. Neurogenesis in adulthood: a possible role in learning. *Trends Cogn. Sci.* 3: 186-92

Gross CG. 2000. Neurogenesis in the adult brain: death of a dogma. *Nat. Rev. Neurosci.* 1: 67-73

Gutman DA, Nemeroff CB. 2003. Persistent central nervous system effects of an adverse early environment: clinical and preclinical studies. *Physiol. Behav.* 79: 471-8

Haley DW, Handmaker NS, Lowe J. 2006. Infant stress reactivity and prenatal alcohol exposure. *Alcohol Clin. Exp. Res.* 30: 2055-64

Hamilton DA, Kodituwakku P, Sutherland RJ, Savage DD. 2003. Children with Fetal Alcohol Syndrome are impaired at place learning but not cued-navigation in a virtual Morris water task. *Behav. Brain Res.* 143: 85-94

Handa RJ, Burgess LH, Kerr JE, O'Keefe JA. 1994. Gonadal steroid hormone receptors and sex differences in the hypothalamo-pituitary-adrenal axis. *Horm. Behav.* 28: 464-76

Hannigan JH, Berman RF, Zajac CS. 1993. Environmental enrichment and the behavioral effects of prenatal exposure to alcohol in rats. *Neurotoxicol. Teratol.* 15: 261-6

Heinz A, Mann K, Weinberger DR, Goldman D. 2001. Serotonergic dysfunction, negative mood states, and response to alcohol. *Alcohol. Clin. Exp. Res.* 25: 487-95

Hellemans KG, Sliwowska JH, Verma P, Weinberg J. 2009. Prenatal alcohol exposure: Fetal programming and later life vulnerability to stress, depression and anxiety disorders. *Neurosci. Biobehav. Rev.*

Herman JP, Cullinan WE. 1997. Neurocircuitry of stress: central control of the hypothalamo-pituitary-adrenocortical axis. *Trends Neurosci.* 20: 78-84

Hofmann CE, Ellis L, Yu WK, Weinberg J. 2007. Hypothalamic-pituitary-adrenal responses to 5-HT1A and 5-HT2A/C agonists are differentially altered in female and male rats prenatally exposed to ethanol. *Alcohol Clin. Exp. Res.* 31: 345-55

Hofmann CE, Patyk IA, Weinberg J. 2005. Prenatal ethanol exposure: sex differences in anxiety and anxiolytic response to a 5-HT1A agonist. *Pharmacol. Biochem. Behav.* 82: 549-58

Hofmann CE, Simms W, Yu WK, Weinberg J. 2002. Prenatal ethanol exposure in rats alters serotonergic-mediated behavioral and physiological function. *Psychopharmacology. (Berl)* 161: 379-86

Holmes MM, Galea LA. 2002. Defensive behavior and hippocampal cell proliferation: differential modulation by naltrexone during stress. *Behav. Neurosci.* 116: 160-8

Holsboer F. 2000. The corticosteroid receptor hypothesis of depression. *Neuropsychopharmacology.* 23: 477-501

Humphrey T. 1967. The development of the human hippocampal fissure. *J. Anat.* 101: 655-76

Iqbal U, Brien JF, Banjanin S, Andrews MH, Matthews SG, Reynolds JN. 2005. Chronic prenatal ethanol exposure alters glucocorticoid signalling in the hippocampus of the postnatal Guinea pig. *J. Neuroendocrinol.* 17: 600-8

Jacobson SW, Bihun JT, Chiodo LM. 1999. Effects of prenatal alcohol and cocaine exposure on infant cortisol levels. *Dev. Psychopathol.* 11: 195-208

Jankord R, Herman JP. 2008. Limbic regulation of hypothalamo-pituitary-adrenocortical function during acute and chronic stress. *Ann. N. Y. Acad. Sci.* 1148: 64-73

Jones KL, Smith DW. 1973. Recognition of the fetal alcohol syndrome in early infancy. *Lancet.* 2: 999-1001

Kaplan MS, Hinds JW. 1977. Neurogenesis in the adult rat: electron microscopic analysis of light radioautographs. *Science.* 197: 1092-4

Kempermann G, Gast D, Gage FH. 2002. Neuroplasticity in old age: sustained fivefold induction of hippocampal neurogenesis by long-term environmental enrichment. *Ann. Neurol.* 52: 135-43

Kempermann G, Kuhn HG, Gage FH. 1997. More hippocampal neurons in adult mice living in an enriched environment. *Nature.* 386: 493-5

Kempermann G, Kuhn HG, Gage FH. 1998. Experience-induced neurogenesis in the senescent dentate gyrus. *J. Neurosci.* 18: 3206-12

Kessler RC. 1997. The effects of stressful life events on depression. *Annu. Rev. Psychol.* 48: 191-214

Kim JA, Druse MJ. 1996. Protective effects of maternal buspirone treatment on serotonin reuptake sites in ethanol-exposed offspring. *Brain Res. Dev. Brain Res.* 92: 190-8

Klintsova AY, Cowell RM, Swain RA, Napper RM, Goodlett CR, Greenough WT. 1998. Therapeutic effects of complex motor training on motor performance deficits induced by neonatal binge-like alcohol exposure in rats . I. Behavioral results. *Brain Res.* 800: 48-61

Kodituwakku PW. 2009. A neurodevelopmental framework for the development of interventions for children with fetal alcohol spectrum disorders. *Alcohol.*

Kolb B, Forgie M, Gibb R, Gorny G, Rowntree S. 1998. Age, experience and the changing brain. *Neurosci. Biobehav. Rev.* 22: 143-59

Konorski J. 1948. Conditioned reflex and neuron organization. Cambridge, UK

Kopelman MD, Thomson AD, Guerrini I, Marshall EJ. 2009. The Korsakoff syndrome: clinical aspects, psychology and treatment. *Alcohol Alcohol.* 44: 148-54

Kurose I, Higuchi H, Kato S, Miura S, Watanabe N, et al. 1997. Oxidative stress on mitochondria and cell membrane of cultured rat hepatocytes and perfused liver exposed to ethanol. *Gastroenterology.* 112: 1331-43

McEwen BS. 2009. The brain is the central organ of stress and adaptation. *Neuroimage.* 47: 911-3

McEwen BS, Magarinos AM. 2001. Stress and hippocampal plasticity: implications for the pathophysiology of affective disorders. *Hum. Psychopharmacol.* 16: S7-S19

McEwen BS, Stellar E. 1993. Stress and the individual. Mechanisms leading to disease. *Arch. Intern. Med.* 153: 2093-101

McEwen BS, Weiss JM, Schwartz LS. 1968. Selective retention of corticosterone by limbic structures in rat brain. *Nature.* 220: 911-2

McEwen BS, Wingfield JC. 2003. The concept of allostasis in biology and biomedicine. *Horm. Behav.* 43: 2-15

McGivern RF, Raum WJ, Handa RJ, Sokol RZ. 1992 Comparision of two week versus one week of prenatal ethanol exposure in the rat on organ weights, sperm count, and onset of puberty. *Neurotoxicol. Teratol.* 14: 351-358

McGivern RF, Yellow SM. 1992 Delayed onset of puberty and subtle alterations in GnRH neuronal morphology in female rats exposed prenatally to ethanol. *Alcohol.* 9:335-40

McKinnon MC, Yucel K, Nazarov A, MacQueen GM. 2009. A meta-analysis examining clinical predictors of hippocampal volume in patients with major depressive disorder. *J. Psychiatry Neurosci.* 34: 41-54

Meaney MJ, Diorio J, Francis D, Weaver S, Yau J, et al. 2000. Postnatal handling increases the expression of cAMP-inducible transcription factors in the rat hippocampus: the effects of thyroid hormones and serotonin. *J. Neurosci.* 20: 3926-35

Meaney MJ, Diorio J, Francis D, Widdowson J, LaPlante P, et al. 1996. Early environmental regulation of forebrain glucocorticoid receptor gene expression: implications for adrenocortical responses to stress. *Dev. Neurosci.* 18: 49-72

Meaney MJ, Szyf M, Seckl JR. 2007. Epigenetic mechanisms of perinatal programming of hypothalamic-pituitary-adrenal function and health. *Trends Mol. Med.* 13: 269-77

Miller G. 2009. The brain collector. *Science.* 324: 1634-6

Miller MW. 1995. Generation of neurons in the rat dentate gyrus and hippocampus: effects of prenatal and postnatal treatment with ethanol. *Alcohol Clin. Exp. Res.* 19: 1500-9

Miller MW. 1996. Effect of early exposure to ethanol on the protein and DNA contents of specific brain regions in the rat. *Brain Res.* 734: 286-94

Mirescu C, Gould E. 2006. Stress and adult neurogenesis. *Hippocampus.* 16: 233-8

Mirescu C, Peters JD, Gould E. 2004. Early life experience alters response of adult neurogenesis to stress. *Nat. Neurosci.* 7: 841-6

Mitchell JB, Iny LJ, Meaney MJ. 1990. The role of serotonin in the development and environmental regulation of type II corticosteroid receptor binding in rat hippocampus. *Brain Res. Dev. Brain Res.* 55: 231-5

Mitchell JJ, Paiva M, Heaton MB. 1999. Vitamin E and beta-carotene protect against ethanol combined with ischemia in an embryonic rat hippocampal culture model of fetal alcohol syndrome. *Neurosci. Lett.* 263: 189-92

Montoliu C, Valles S, Renau-Piqueras J, Guerri C. 1994. Ethanol-induced oxygen radical formation and lipid peroxidation in rat brain: effect of chronic alcohol consumption. *J. Neurochem.* 63: 1855-62

Morris R. 2007. Stress and the Hippocampus. In *The Hippocampus Book*, ed. MR Andersen P., Amaral D., Bliss T., O'Keefe J., pp. pp.751-68. New York: Oxford University Press

Morris RG, Garrud P, Rawlins JN, O'Keefe J. 1982. Place navigation impaired in rats with hippocampal lesions. *Nature.* 297: 681-3

Nestler EJ, Barrot M, DiLeone RJ, Eisch AJ, Gold SJ, Monteggia LM. 2002. Neurobiology of depression. *Neuron.* 34: 13-25

Nilsson M, Perfilieva E, Johansson U, Orwar O, Eriksson PS. 1999. Enriched environment increases neurogenesis in the adult rat dentate gyrus and improves spatial memory. *J. Neurobiol.* 39: 569-78

O'Connor MJ, Kasari C. 2000. Prenatal alcohol exposure and depressive features in children. *Alcohol Clin. Exp. Res.* 24: 1084-92

O'Connor MJ, Paley B. 2006. The relationship of prenatal alcohol exposure and the postnatal environment to child depressive symptoms. *J. Pediatr. Psychol.* 31: 50-64

Oitzl MS, Champagne DL, van der Veen R, de Kloet ER. 2009. Brain development under stress: Hypotheses of glucocorticoid actions revisited. *Neurosci. Biobehav. Rev.*

O'Keefe J. 1993. Hippocampus, theta, and spatial memory. *Curr. Opin. Neurobiol.* 3: 917-24

Olsen H, Morse B, Huffine C. 1998. Development and Psychopathology: Fetal Alcohol Syndrome and Related Conditions. *Semin. Clin. Neuropsychiatry.* 3: 262-84

Olson HC, Morse BA, Huffine C. 1998. Development and Psychopathology: Fetal Alcohol Syndrome and Related Conditions. *Semin. Clin. Neuropsychiatry.* 3: 262-84

Olson HC, Oti R, Gelo J, Beck S. 2009. "Family matters:" fetal alcohol spectrum disorders and the family. *Dev. Disabil. Res. Rev.* 15: 235-49

Olton DS. 1977a. The function of septo-hippocampal connections in spatially organized behaviour. *Ciba Found. Symp*: 327-49

Olton DS. 1977b. Spatial memory. *Sci. Am.* 236: 82-4, 9-94, 6, 8

Opitz B, Mothes HK, Clausing P. 1997. Effects of prenatal ethanol exposure and early experience on radial maze performance and conditioned taste aversion in mice. *Neurotoxicol. Teratol.* 19: 185-90

Osborne GL, Caul WF, Fernandez K. 1980. Behavioral effects of prenatal ethanol exposure and differential early experience in rats. *Pharmacol. Biochem. Behav.* 12: 393-401

Peadon E, Rhys-Jones B, Bower C, Elliott EJ. 2009. Systematic review of interventions for children with Fetal Alcohol Spectrum Disorders. *BMC Pediatr.* 9: 35

Per Andersen RM, David Amaral, Tim Bliss, and John O'Keefe. 2007. Historical perspective: proposed functions, biological characteristics, and neurobiological models of the hippocampus. In *The hippocampus book*, ed. RM Per Andersen, David Amaral, Tim Bliss, and John O'Keefe, pp. p.9. New York: Oxford University Press

Pham K, Nacher J, Hof PR, McEwen BS. 2003. Repeated restraint stress suppresses neurogenesis and induces biphasic PSA-NCAM expression in the adult rat dentate gyrus. *Eur. J. Neurosci.* 17: 879-86

Phillips DI, Barker DJ, Fall CH, Seckl JR, Whorwood CB, et al. 1998. Elevated plasma cortisol concentrations: a link between low birth weight and the insulin resistance syndrome? *J. Clin. Endocrinol. Metab.* 83: 757-60

Phillips DI, Walker BR, Reynolds RM, Flanagan DE, Wood PJ, et al. 2000. Low birth weight predicts elevated plasma cortisol concentrations in adults from 3 populations. *Hypertension.* 35: 1301-6

Plato (reprint 1952). Laws.

Ponnappa BC, Rubin E. 2000. Modeling alcohol's effects on organs in animal models. *Alcohol. Res. Health.* 24: 93-104

Pryce CR, Ruedi-Bettschen D, Dettling AC, Weston A, Russig H, et al. 2005. Long-term effects of early-life environmental manipulations in rodents and primates: Potential animal models in depression research. *Neurosci. Biobehav. Rev.* 29: 649-74

Ramsay DS, Bendersky MI, Lewis M. 1996. Effect of prenatal alcohol and cigarette exposure on two- and six-month-old infants' adrenocortical reactivity to stress. *J. Pediatr. Psychol.* 21: 833-40

Rathbun W, Druse MJ. 1985. Dopamine, serotonin, and acid metabolites in brain regions from the developing offspring of ethanol-treated rats. *J. Neurochem.* 44: 57-62

Redila VA, Olson AK, Swann SE, Mohades G, Webber AJ, et al. 2006. Hippocampal cell proliferation is reduced following prenatal ethanol exposure but can be rescued with voluntary exercise. *Hippocampus.* 16: 305-11

Reul JM, van den Bosch FR, de Kloet ER. 1987. Relative occupation of type-I and type-II corticosteroid receptors in rat brain following stress and dexamethasone treatment: functional implications. *J. Endocrinol.* 115: 459-67

Richardson DP, Byrnes ML, Brien JF, Reynolds JN, Dringenberg HC. 2002. Impaired acquisition in the water maze and hippocampal long-term potentiation after chronic prenatal ethanol exposure in the guinea-pig. *Eur. J. Neurosci.* 16: 1593-8

Riikonen R, Salonen I, Partanen K, Verho S. 1999. Brain perfusion SPECT and MRI in foetal alcohol syndrome. *Dev. Med. Child Neurol.* 41: 652-9

Riikonen RS, Nokelainen P, Valkonen K, Kolehmainen AI, Kumpulainen KI, et al. 2005. Deep serotonergic and dopaminergic structures in fetal alcoholic syndrome: a study with nor-beta-CIT-single-photon emission computed tomography and magnetic resonance imaging volumetry. *Biol. Psychiatry.* 57: 1565-72

Riley EP, Barron S, Hannigan J. 1986. Response inhibition deficits following prenatal alcohol exposure: a comparision to the effects of hippocampal lesions in rats. In *Alcohol and brain development.*, ed. J West, pp. p.71-102. New York: Oxford University Press

Rogers RL, Meyer JS, Mortel KF. 1990. After reaching retirement age physical activity sustains cerebral perfusion and cognition. *J. Am. Geriatr. Soc.* 38: 123-8

Romero LM, Dickens MJ, Cyr NE. 2009. The Reactive Scope Model - a new model integrating homeostasis, allostasis, and stress. *Horm. Behav.* 55: 375-89

Rosenzweig MR. 1996. Aspects of the search for neural mechanisms of memory. *Annu. Rev. Psychol.* 47: 1-32

Sapolsky RM. 1992. Do glucocorticoid concentrations rise with age in the rat? *Neurobiol. Aging.* 13: 171-4

Sapolsky RM. 1997. McEwen-Induced Modulation of Endocrine History: A Partial Review. *Stress.* 2: 1-12

Taylor AN, Branch BJ, Liu SH, Kokka N. 1982. Long-term effects of fetal ethanol exposure on pituitary-adrenal response to stress. *Pharmacol. Biochem. Behav.* 16: 585-9

Taylor AN, Branch BJ, Nelson LR, Lane LA, Poland RE. 1986. Prenatal ethanol and ontogeny of pituitary-adrenal responses to ethanol and morphine. *Alcohol.* 3: 255-9

Taylor AN, Nelson LR, Branch BJ, Kokka N, Poland RE. 1984. Altered stress responsiveness in adult rats exposed to ethanol in utero: neuroendocrine mechanisms. *Ciba Found Symp.* 105: 47-65

Thase ME. 2006. Depression and sleep: pathophysiology and treatment. *Dialogues Clin. Neurosci.* 8: 217-26

Tyrer P, Baldwin D. 2006. Generalised anxiety disorder. *Lancet.* 368: 2156-66

Uecker A, Nadel L. 1996. Spatial locations gone awry: object and spatial memory deficits in children with fetal alcohol syndrome. *Neuropsychologia.* 34: 209-23

Uecker A, Nadel L. 1998. Spatial but not object memory impairments in children with fetal alcohol syndrome. *Am. J. Ment. Retard.* 103: 12-8

Van Gijn J. 2001. The hidden structure: A scientific biography of Camillo Golgi. By Paolo Mazzarello -Book review. *The New England Journal of Medicine.* 344: 1102

van Praag H. 2008. Neurogenesis and exercise: past and future directions. *Neuromolecular Med.* 10: 128-40

van Praag H, Christie BR, Sejnowski TJ, Gage FH. 1999a. Running enhances neurogenesis, learning, and long-term potentiation in mice. *Proc. Natl. Acad. Sci. U. S. A.* 96: 13427-31

van Praag H, Kempermann G, Gage FH. 1999b. Running increases cell proliferation and neurogenesis in the adult mouse dentate gyrus. *Nat. Neurosci.* 2: 266-70

Viau V, Meaney MJ. 1991. Variations in the hypothalamic-pituitary-adrenal response to stress during the estrous cycle in the rat. *Endocrinology.* 129: 2503-11

Vieau, D., Sebaai, N., Leonhardt, M., Dutriez-Casteloot, I., Molendi-Coste, O., Laborie, C., Breton, C., Deloof, S., Lesage, J., 2007. HPA axis programming by maternal undernutrition in the male rat offspring. *Psychoneuroendocrinology* 32 (Suppl.1), S16–S20

Vink J, Auth J, Abebe DT, Brenneman DE, Spong CY. 2005. Novel peptides prevent alcohol-induced spatial learning deficits and proinflammatory cytokine release in a mouse model of fetal alcohol syndrome. *Am. J. Obstet. Gynecol.* 193: 825-9

Waddell BJ, Benediktsson R, Brown RW, Seckl JR. 1998. Tissue-specific messenger ribonucleic acid expression of 11beta-hydroxysteroid dehydrogenase types 1 and 2 and the glucocorticoid receptor within rat placenta suggests exquisite local control of glucocorticoid action. *Endocrinology.* 139: 1517-23

Wainwright PE, Levesque S, Krempulec L, Bulman-Fleming B, McCutcheon D. 1993. Effects of environmental enrichment on cortical depth and Morris-maze performance in B6D2F2 mice exposed prenatally to ethanol. *Neurotoxicol. Teratol.* 15: 11-20

Warren, KR., and Foudin, LL. 2001. Alcohol related birth defects—The past, present, and future. *Alcohol Research & Health.*25(3):153–158

Walsberg GE. 2003. How useful is energy balance as a overall index of stress in animals? *Horm. Behav.* 43: 16-7; discussion 28-30

Weiler IJ, Hawrylak N, Greenough WT. 1995. Morphogenesis in memory formation: synaptic and cellular mechanisms. *Behav. Brain Res.* 66: 1-6

Weinberg J. 1984. Nutritional issues in perinatal alcohol exposure. *Neurobehav. Toxicol. Teratol.* 6: 261-9

Weinberg J. 1988. Hyperresponsiveness to stress: differential effects of prenatal ethanol on males and females. *Alcohol Clin. Exp. Res.* 12: 647-52

Weinberg J. 1992. Prenatal ethanol effects: sex differences in offspring stress responsiveness. *Alcohol.* 9: 219-23

Weinberg J, Sliwowska JH, Lan N, Hellemans KG. 2008. Prenatal alcohol exposure: foetal programming, the hypothalamic-pituitary-adrenal axis and sex differences in outcome. *J. Neuroendocrinol.* 20: 470-88

Welberg LA, Seckl JR. 2001. Prenatal stress, glucocorticoids and the programming of the brain. *J. Neuroendocrinol.* 13: 113-28

West JR, Goodlett CR. 1990. Teratogenic effects of alcohol on brain development. *Ann. Med.* 22: 319-25

West JR, Hamre KM, Cassell MD. 1986. Effects of ethanol exposure during the third trimester equivalent on neuron number in rat hippocampus and dentate gyrus. *Alcohol Clin. Exp. Res.* 10: 190-7

West JR, Hodges CA, Black AC, Jr. 1981. Prenatal exposure to ethanol alters the organization of hippocampal mossy fibers in rats. *Science.* 211: 957-9

West JR, Kelly SJ, Pierce DR. 1987. Severity of alcohol-induced deficits in rats during the third trimester equivalent is determined by the pattern of exposure. *Alcohol Alcohol Suppl.* 1: 461-5

Whitaker-Azmitia PM, Druse M, Walker P, Lauder JM. 1996. Serotonin as a developmental signal. *Behav. Brain Res.* 73: 19-29

White PC, Mune T, Rogerson FM, Kayes KM, Agarwal AK. 1997. 11 beta-Hydroxysteroid dehydrogenase and its role in the syndrome of apparent mineralocorticoid excess. *Pediatr. Res.* 41: 25-9

Willford JA, Richardson GA, Leech SL, Day NL. 2004. Verbal and visuospatial learning and memory function in children with moderate prenatal alcohol exposure. *Alcohol Clin. Exp. Res.* 28: 497-507

Wilson ME, Handa RJ.1997.Gonadotropin secretion in infantile rats exposed to ethanol in utero. *Alcohol.* 14:497-501

Winter B, Breitenstein C, Mooren FC, Voelker K, Fobker M, et al. 2007. High impact running improves learning. *Neurobiol. Learn. Mem.* 87: 597-609

Yamashita F, Lan N, Yu W, Ellis L, AG H, Weinberg J. 2004. Role of estradiol in stress hyperresponsiveness seen in female rats preanatally exposed to ethanol. *Neurotoxicol. Teratol.* 26: 502

Zhang X, Sliwowska JH, Weinberg J. 2005. Prenatal alcohol exposure and fetal programming: effects on neuroendocrine and immune function. *Exp. Biol. Med. (Maywood)* 230: 376-88

Zhou FC, Sari Y, Powrozek TA. 2005. Fetal alcohol exposure reduces serotonin innervation and compromises development of the forebrain along the serotonergic pathway. *Alcohol Clin. Exp. Res.* 29: 141-9

Zhou FC, Sari Y, Powrozek TA, Spong CY. 2004. A neuroprotective peptide antagonizes fetal alcohol exposure-compromised brain growth. *J. Mol. Neurosci.* 24: 189-99

Zhou FC, Sari Y, Zhang JK, Goodlett CR, Li T. 2001. Prenatal alcohol exposure retards the migration and development of serotonin neurons in fetal C57BL mice. *Brain Res. Dev. Brain Res.* 126: 147-55

Index

C

D

E

F

G

H

I

S

T